Lived Realities of Solo Motherhood, Donor Conception and Medically Assisted Reproduction

Emerald Studies in Reproduction, Culture and Society

Series Editors: Petra Nordqvist, Manchester University, UK and Nicky Hudson, De Montfort University, UK

This book series brings together scholars from across the social sciences and humanities who are working in the broad field of human reproduction. Reproduction is a growing field of interest in the UK and internationally, and this series publishes work from across the lifecycle of reproduction addressing issues such as conception, contraception, abortion, pregnancy, birth, infertility, pre and postnatal care, pre-natal screen and testing, IVF, prenatal genetic diagnosis, mitochondrial donation, surrogacy, adoption, reproductive donation, family-making and more. Books in this series will focus on the social, cultural, material, legal, historical and political aspects of human reproduction, encouraging work from early career researchers as well as established scholars. The series includes monographs, edited collections and shortform books (between 20 and 50,000 words). Contributors use the latest conceptual, methodological and theoretical developments to enhance and develop current thinking about human reproduction and its significance for understanding wider social practices and processes.

Published Titles in This Series

Egg Freezing, Fertility and Reproductive Choice
Authored by *Kylie Baldwin*

The Cryopolitics of Reproduction on Ice: A New Scandinavian Ice Age
Authored by *Charlotte Kr_Løkke, Thomas Søbirk Petersen, Janne Rothmar Herrmann, Anna Sofie Bach, Stine Willum Adrian, Rune Klingenberg and Michael Nebeling Petersen*

Voluntary and Involuntary Childlessness
Edited by *Natalie Sappleton*

Lived Realities of Solo Motherhood, Donor Conception and Medically Assisted Reproduction

By

TINE RAVN

Aarhus University, Denmark

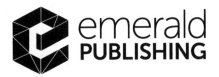

United Kingdom – North America – Japan – India – Malaysia – China

Emerald Publishing Limited
Howard House, Wagon Lane, Bingley BD16 1WA, UK

First edition 2021

Reprints and permissions service
Contact: permissions@emeraldinsight.com

British Library Cataloguing in Publication Data
A catalogue record for this book is available from the British Library

ISBN: 978-1-83909-116-2 (Print)
ISBN: 978-1-83909-115-5 (Online)
ISBN: 978-1-83909-117-9 (Epub)

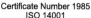

ISOQAR certified
Management System,
awarded to Emerald
for adherence to
Environmental
standard
ISO 14001:2004.

Certificate Number 1985
ISO 14001

INVESTOR IN PEOPLE

To all the women who participated in this study

Table of Contents

List of Figures and Tables

About the Author

Tine Ravn, PhD, is an Assistant Professor at the Danish Centre for Studies in Research and Research Policy, Department of Political Science at Aarhus University. Her work broadly concerns the relationship between science and society with a particular focus on the social, legislative and ethical aspects of medical biotechnologies, research integrity/research ethics and public engagement with science and technology. She has a particular interest in assisted reproductive technologies (ARTs), solo motherhood, kinship and identity. Together with good colleagues, she has co-authored the book *Social Theory: a Textbook* published by Routledge.

Acknowledgements

Overall, this is a book about life trajectories and how one is to navigate them, when no well-defined maps of life are available; when there is only the most basic coordinates and greater landmarks but no master cartography to be found. Some routes are, however, more well travelled than others. Embarking upon solo motherhood through donor conception as a particular route to motherhood is not one such well-travelled path and new strategies for and in life have to be explored. I am exceedingly grateful to the women in this study, for choosing to share their life stories with me and for giving me an insight into the lived realities of solo motherhood through donor conception. Their honest, personal, detailed and vivid narratives have formed the basis of this book and they deserve to be read in full with all the depth, complexity and richness that characterize them. Still, I hope my selection, analysis and representation will do them justice and also demonstrate individual life story integrity and profundity.

I would also like to thank Lone Schmidt, Maria Salomon and Karin Erb for lending their vast knowledge and expertise on this field, and for their readiness to answer my many questions and requests. In August 2015, I spent two days at the Fertility Clinic at Arhus University Hospital. I am very grateful to all the employees at the clinic for letting me be part of their professional daily routines and for taking time out of their busy schedule to acquaint me with the various fertility procedures and practices. I owe special thanks to Hans Jakob Ingerslev for arranging and coordinating my stay at the clinic. I would also like to thank the many fertility clinics across Denmark who helped me disseminate knowledge about this study. These are the public fertility clinics located in Odense, Skejby (Aarhus), Dronninglund, Randers and Greater Copenhagen. The private clinics are The Danish Fertility Clinic Copenhagen (Danfert), Stork Clinic in Copenhagen and Fertility Clinic IVF-SYD in Fredericia. I would also like to thank Signe Fjord and the online forum for single women by choice (SEM) for helping me disseminate information about this study through their online resources.

This book builds on the study on solo motherhood conducted as part of my PhD and the monograph 'Strategies for Life – Lived Realities of Solo Motherhood, Kinship and Medically Assisted Reproduction'. I am grateful to the Aarhus BSS Graduate School for funding this work based at the Danish Centre for Studies in Research and Research Policy (CFA) at Aarhus University. It is an absolute pleasure to be part of the Centre and its vibrant, interdisciplinary and convivial atmosphere. I would like to thank all of my current and former colleagues for adding to this positive setting and for all the support, valuable collaborations, inspirational academic presentations, discussions and social events that have shaped my daily work life and formed my professional identity.

A very special thanks goes to my former PhD supervisors Mads P. Sørensen and Trine Lund Thomsen for all of their vast support, mentoring and knowledgeable, insightful and experienced guidance which have been a valuable and essential source of inspiration and encouragement for developing the present work. I would also particularly like to thank Niels Mejlgaard, Carter Bloch, Lise Degn, Sanne Haase, Mathias Wullum Nielsen, Jane Frølund Irming, Heidi Skovgaard Pedersen, Catherine McDonald, Morten Suusgaard, Sigrid Dohn Raunkjær, Christoffer Andresen, Emil Madsen, Jens Viuff Ludvigsen and Malene Christensen for all their support, feedback and cheering, and for various forms of invaluable assistance from moral support over reference and language editing to transcribing interviews during the process of research and writing.

I would also very much like to thank the series editors Petra Nordqvist and Nicky Hudson for their support and their perceptive and constructive feedback. I would also very much like to thank senior publishers Kim Chadwick and Jen McCall for proficiently steering the book through the stages of publishing and the first-rate editorial and production team who assisted this process, including Pavithra Muthu, Dheebika Veerasamy, Abi Masha, Harriet Notman, Nagaruru Balaji Sai and Carys Morley.

As part of the research, I was so fortunate to be able to visit The Centre for Family Research at the University of Cambridge for a month in 2016. I am very grateful to Centre Director Susan Golombok for the invitation to visit this vibrant, inspiring and academically outstanding environment. I would like to thank all employees for their very welcoming and positive approach and particularly to administrator Abby Scott. I owe a special thanks to Susanna Graham for making the stay possible and for sharing with me her unrivalled insights and expertise within the field. Susanna's wise comments, encouragement and support have been of vital importance for this study. I not only consider her to be a valued collaborator but also an appreciated friend and I hope to be able to expand our collaboration in the future.

At last I would like to thank my closest family and friends for their great and treasured support during this prolonged process. It must seem as if I have been researching and writing this book forever, and I am very grateful for their constant caring and encouragement.

First and foremost, I am exceedingly grateful for my partner Stefan, our children Selma and Theo and their unconditional love and support. I do not know how I would have found my way through this project – and through life in general – if it had not been for them. They are truly the ones who provide meaning and direction in my life and words cannot express how privileged I feel being able to share and explore life with them.

Introduction: Puzzling Paradoxes of Nature versus Nurture

> Love is what ties a family together. Comfort. So it doesn't have to be the family tree in perfectly straight, beautiful rows, dak dak. There can be a few offshoots here and there, things that aren't connected purely genetically.
>
> —Charlotte (Physiotherapist, in treatment with IUI-D)

In the intersecting contexts of novel technologies and sociocultural transformations, new options for parenthood and family formation have emerged, fostering a diversity in kinship practices and revised understandings of relatedness and familial ties. New meanings are ascribed to biogenetic relations while they also continue to form an important part of contemporary family life (Franklin, 2013b; Nordqvist, 2017). Likewise, the meaning of motherhood has branched out from biological and social motherhood to include notions of genetic, gestational and epigenetic motherhood (Hertz, 2021; Payne, 2016). Single women, like Charlotte in the introductory epigraph, constitute a growing group of women who pursue the technological options available and choose to embark upon solo motherhood through the means of medically assisted reproduction (MAR). Based on an interdisciplinary approach and an array of empirical data, this book asks and seeks to answer questions such as: How do single women experience the choice of contemplating solo motherhood and how do they rationalize and normalize this choice? How do processes of fertility treatment influence the life planning/biographical revisions of solo mothers and how does the interplay of biogenetic and social ties influence family and kinship conceptions and actual family constructions?

Hence, this book explores the lived realities of embarking upon solo motherhood and the process of undergoing fertility treatment. It provides insights into the complexities related to forming donor-conceived families through MAR, and it explores to which extent such technological possibilities in combination with sociocultural developments and the production of new legislation have challenged traditional ideas about kinship and facilitated the increase in 'new' kinship and family practices. The book explores personal narratives to uncover how established, sociocultural narratives are adopted, negotiated and transformed in the processes of decision-making, fertility treatment and in the building of solo mother families.

Lived Realities of Solo Motherhood, Donor Conception
and Medically Assisted Reproduction, 1–13
Copyright © 2021 Tine Ravn
Published under exclusive licence by Emerald Publishing Limited
doi:10.1108/978-1-83909-115-520211001

This introductory chapter sets the stage for the remaining book. It frames the rise of new family forms by means of assisted reproduction, and it presents a series of paradoxes that characterize the developments and expansion of MAR in a context of human reproduction and donor conception. These paradoxes all revolve around reproductive technologies and their uncanny ability to both mirror and destabilize our 'natural' assumptions about reproduction, family and kinship (Franklin, 2013a). Originally designed to help heterosexual couples build nuclear families, assisted reproductive technologies (ARTs) are now helping in bringing about new types of families – such as the solo mother family (Golombok, 2015). In the wake of these developments, the introduction asks how we define, legislate and practice relatedness now that human procreation has ceased to depend on sexual relations, and distinctions between biogenetic and social aspects of family formation have been weakened. By addressing the culture and nature (nurture and nature) distinction and its transgression – a recurring motif in this book – the introduction queries and outlines how such paradoxical pairs are subject to interpretation, normalization and malleability in relation to the concept of the solo mother family.

MAR and the Formation of Solo Mother Families

> The bio-cultural impacts of ARTs is not likely to decrease any time soon – on the contrary, reproductive technologies are likely to continue having a major impact on how we understand not only reproductive practices and rights, but also human life as such.
> –Jenny (2013, p. 241)

During the past three decades, advances within MAR have led to its rapid development and expansion and the various reproductive technologies and techniques available have increasingly become a widespread and routinized means of alleviating infertility and assisting with conception. Yet, as Sarah Franklin argues, the 'technologization of reproduction is both ordinary and curious' (2013a, p. 1) in the sense of becoming ever more familiar, while simultaneously possessing a number of paradoxical features by both imitating and destabilizing 'natural' forms of procreation and kinship relations, and therefore transgressing taken-for-granted dichotomies such as that found between nature and culture (Franklin, 2013a; Inhorn and Birenbaum-Carmeli, 2008; McKinnon, 2015).

While ARTs were initially developed and designed with the purpose of helping heterosexual couples build nuclear families comprising a mother, father and one or more biological children, 'new families' (Golombok, 2015, p. 3) such as lesbian mother families, gay father families and solo mother families are increasingly being formed via the utilization of assisted reproduction. These novel ways of 'doing' family – novel in the sense that they did not exist or were unknown to society until late in the twentieth century - create new relationship forms that often involve known or unknown 'reproductive others' (Freeman, 2014, p. 2) in the form of eggs, sperm and embryo donors and/or surrogates (Mckinnon, 2015; Golombok, 2015).

'Single mothers by choice' (SMC), 'solo mothers' or 'choice mothers' are women who intentionally choose to conceive a child and act as the sole parent. The 'by choice' aspect constitutes the key defining element which sets this group of women apart from mothers who, for instance, have become single-after-the-fact due to factors such as divorce, separation or the death of a partner (Golombok, 2015; Graham and Braverman, 2012). The means of becoming a single mother by choice varies and where some choose to adopt or become pregnant through a sexual encounter, others make use of assisted reproductive procedures (IUI-D and ART) with a known or un-known donor. The latter approach seems to be the most common route to motherhood (Golombok, 2015). The interviewed women in this book have all embarked upon solo motherhood through MAR.

The possibilities provided or enhanced by reproductive technologies have raised a number of legal, sociocultural and ethical issues and provoked responses regarding their ramifications whilst simultaneously shaping and being shaped by the societal and individual contexts in which they are situated and practiced (Inhorn and Birenbaum-Carmeli, 2008; Freeman, 2014). How are we therefore to legislate, define and practice relatedness when the distinction between biogenetic and social aspects of family formation and kinship-making are no longer as connected to nature as previously presumed? As Charis Thompson states in this regard, 'assisted reproductive technologies demand as much social as techno-logical innovation to make sense of the biological and social relationships that ARTs forge and deny' (2005, p. 5). In this regard, Nordqvist and Smart argue that families with donor-conceived children 'are at the forefront of a modern debate about the conflicting significance of nature versus nature' (2014, p. 150) in defining and redefining the meaning of genetic and social relatedness.

A number of puzzling paradoxes seem to characterize the developments and expansion of MAR. These paradoxes revolve around the double feature of imitating and destabilizing 'natural' forms of procreation and kinship relations in diversifying hitherto unquestioned binaries, such as nature/culture, biology/sociality and sex/procreation (Franklin, 2013a; McKinnon, 2015). This book explores the empirical manifestations of such paradoxes within a particular situated context and provide in-depth understandings of solo motherhood through assisted reproduction as a specific case to understand the lived realities and experiences of creating donor-conceived families.

At its heart, the book is engaged with how biogenetic and social connections (nature-culture) are defined and given meaning when family and kinship relations are literally and actively created by those involved in them. It is explored through the women's strategies for creating life through assisted reproduction and building life as a solo mother, for instance in terms of the strategies used to motivate the decision to parent alone and the strategies invoked to claim an own child through the use of donor conception. The book seeks to provide new understandings of how single women 'do' family, identity and kinship and how the choice to create life as a solo mother is continuously rationalized and normalized. While the decision – and the child's conception – is for life, the book shows that the considerations and understandings of what is 'given' and what is 'made' in terms of establishing kinship and family relations (Carsten, 2004, p. 9), are dynamic and variant and help to shape familial narratives of e.g. mother–child relations and donor–donor sibling relations.

The (re)configuration of the nature/culture distinction – with regard to normalization processes vis-à-vis technological advances – constitutes a main perspective in this book's exploration of the ramifications of assisted reproduction, as these technologies may possibly incur further redefinitions of our understandings of 'normal' procreation, 'normal' family formation and 'normal' motherhood, among others. There have always been certain prevalent ideas – about what can and cannot be conceived of as 'natural' states and ways of life in the context of human beings – and 'with time, it is striking how different the line between the natural and the unnatural has been drawn' (Balling and Lippert-Rasmussen, 2006, p. 19). In this regard, biotechnological innovations represent ongoing possibilities which challenge our perceptions of the notion of 'natural' (p. 20). In this regard, ARTs constitute a normative as well as moral and ethical field of research, as they bring essential issues into play and transgress a number of more or less established concepts within modernity in collapsing 'the separations between nature and culture, home and work, love and money, the domestic and the economic' (McKinnon, 2015, p. 477). Moreover, the increasingly fluid boundary between nature and culture has spurred legal and political efforts to re-establish and define this line in new ways, through processes of regulation (Lemke, 2009). While the implications of innovations within the field of MAR (e.g. new techniques within embryo research and gamete donation) have yielded policy actions and legal responses internationally from the 1980s onwards, the issues of when a life begins, of 'natural' family structures and access to treatment and of women's reproductive rights, among others, have been managed and regulated in diverse ways across the world (Cooper and Waldby, 2014, p. 46).

Legal MAR Framework

In 2000, Australia was one of the first countries to grant single women access to ARTs. Other countries have then followed. For instance, in the UK, single women gained legislative right to use ARTs in 2008 (Golombok, 2020, pp. 145–146). Since 2009, the introduction of ART legislation has expanded and, today, almost all European countries have implemented some kind of ART legislation. Specific legislation do however differ among countries, for instance in relation to ART procedures such as embryo freezing and egg donation, donor anonymity and access criteria. The European countries are for instance divided in whether they grant single women access to ARTs (Präg and Mills, 2017; ESHRE, 2017; see Chapter 3 for details).

Within the Danish context, in which the study is situated, a complex set of regulations and legislation have continuously been produced. Two pieces of legislation in particular constitute a legislative framework for this book. In

January 2007, single and lesbian women in Denmark gained the legal right to assisted reproduction, permitting doctors in both the public and private health care system to offer assisted reproduction to all women, regardless of marital status or sexual orientation. Prior to this amendment, single and lesbian women were only able to make use of donor insemination (DI) in private midwifery clinics and were thus not able to access any kind of medical care which essentially excluded the group of women who needed medical infertility assistance.

In addition to the legislation introduced in 2007, the Danish regulation on sperm donation was revised in 2012 to introduce a new identity-release donor option, in contrast to the sole existing option allowing only anonymous sperm donation to be used in medically run clinics. In the wake of increasing debate and research into 'donor disclosure' (i.e. access to information about one's paternal genetic inheritance), recent years have seen an introduction of identity-release donors in countries such as the UK, New Zealand, Austria and Switzerland. The Nordic countries of Sweden, Norway and Finland have also implemented legislation that makes identity-release donation the only option (Lampic et al., 2014; Blyth and Frith, 2009, p. 177). The distinctive Danish two-way donor system allows for a comparison of rationales for choosing different donor programmes, including underlying perceptions of distinctions between nature and nurture and likewise between kin and non-kin relations, for instance (see Chapter 7). As mentioned earlier and contrary to initial objectives, reproductive technologies have paradoxically destabilized ideas about 'natural' kinship and family relations and while they are still based on 'biological substances and practices', they have nonetheless triggered a questioning of important and non-important biological claims in kinship making (McKinnon, 2015, p. 464). In general, a number of puzzling paradoxes seem not only to characterize the innovations of reproductive technologies but also to map onto the choice of embarking upon solo motherhood.

The Expansion of Assisted Reproduction

It is estimated that around 9 million babies have been born worldwide by means of ARTs. In this regard, Europe takes a leading position in ART with the initiation of around 50% of the reported treatment cycles. Per million population, Belgium and the Nordic countries have the highest ART availability when it comes to cycles (ESHRE, 2020). In addition to helping to create new families and assisting heterosexual couples to become parents, advances in genetic screening and mitochondrial donation have enabled people in risk of passing on a serious mitochondrial disease onto their children to become parents without this risk. Egg donation technologies have furthermore enabled some women to respond to age-related fertility and conceive a child by means of an egg donor (Baldwin, 2019; Hertz, 2021).

Denmark takes a leading position with being one of the countries in the world where most children are born through MAR (Kroløkke et al., 2019). Hence, the use of MAR has become particularly prevalent in Denmark with around 10.5% (2019 estimate) of the children born in a given year being conceived via assisted reproduction. This corresponds to 6.429 of the total number of children estimated to be born in 2019. Against this, it is estimated that 767 of these children will be born to Danish single women without a partner (Danish Fertility Society, 2020a).

The new possibilities for family formation provided by the 2007 change in access has, among other factors, influenced the growing trend of forming solo mother families largely because of the increase in national treatment options (i.e. availability of treatment in public clinics and access to ART treatment). Data on fertility treatment for the entire health sector are reported on a regularly basis through an established reporting system, however with more complete and precise data from 2013 onwards. Hence, it is estimated that 489 children were born through assisted reproduction to Danish women without a partner in 2013. A number that increased to an estimated number of 709 children in 2018. It is more difficult to assess the number of children born prior to 2013 to single women, but based on the data available, it is estimated that around 300–400 children were born annually in the years before 2012 (Danish Fertility Society, 2020, Erb, expert interview). If we look at the total number of women without a partner embarking upon assisted reproduction, we see that a total of 1,129 single women initiated fertility treatment in 2011 compared to 1,870 women in 2019 (see Fig. 1.1). While increases in percentages are almost similar for both groups,

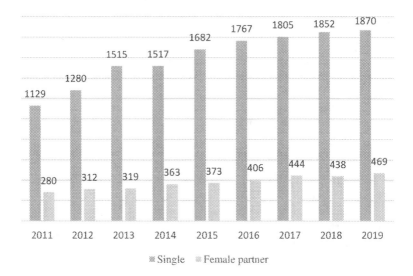

Fig. 1.1.   Total Number of Danish Single Women and Women with Female Partners in Fertility Treatment, 2011–2019. *Note:* If a woman has been undergoing fertility treatment for more than a year, she will figure in both years. Women are defined by their civil registration number. Treatments include IVF, ICSI, Oocyte donation, IUI (D), IUI (H) and Frozen Embryo Replacement (FER). *Source:* The table is constructed based on numbers provided by the Danish Health Data Authority (data from the Danish IVF-Register)

a greater number of single women choose to initiate treatment compared to the group of women with a female partner.

Puzzling Paradoxes

In 1978 on July 25, a baby girl called Louise Brown was born at Oldham General Infirmary in Great Britain. In many ways, this particular birth signified the crucial beginning of a reproductive revolution in which human procreation ceased to depend on sexual relations and 'the natural facts' of sexual reproduction (Franklin, 2008, p. 148), and enabled conception to take place outside of the body (Melhuus, 2012, p. 4). Hence, Louise Brown was born as the world's first 'test-tube' baby with the help of in vitro fertilization (IVF). IVF is a technique in which eggs and sperm are fertilized outside the body (in vitro) whereupon the fertilized embryos are transferred back into the uterus. IVF is one of the most familiar of many techniques labelled 'assisted reproductive technologies' (ARTs) (Franklin, 2008; Inhorn and Birenbaum-Carmeli, 2008). ART is a term that refers to 'all treatments or procedures that include the in vitro handling of both human oocytes and sperm, or embryos, for the purpose of establishing a pregnancy'. Moreover, the collective term 'medically assisted reproduction' (MAR) includes ART treatments *and* intrauterine insemination (IUI) with partner sperm (IUI-H) or donor sperm (IUI-D) (Zegers-Hochschild et al., 2009, p. 2685; Zegers-Hochschild et al., 2017).

Donor insemination is the oldest technique when it comes to 'the new technologies of reproduction' with the first successfully known case dating back to 1884. However, it did not receive full attention until the 1970s and 1980s with the rise of technologies such as IVF (Haimes and Daniels, 1998, p. 1). For single women wishing to have a child on their own, donor insemination (IUI-D) is the standard technology applied unless IVF treatment is required due to infertility issues. IUI is sometimes described as a more 'low tech' procedure, whereas procedures such as IVF are referred to as 'high tech' since they require to a greater extent 'technical competence and sophisticated technological equipment' (Blyth and Landau, 2003, p. 10).[1]

The 9 million babies that have been born worldwide by means of ARTs, indicates 'the fundamental bio-cultural transformation' which has followed in the wake of the realization of IVF and which has led to comprehensive developments within the bio- and genetic technologies (Jenny, 2013, p. 236).

> Not only has the ability directly to manipulate human fertilization and embryology altered the meaning of 'the facts of life'; it has also challenged the idea that biology provides a 'base' on which society is built.
>
> –Franklin (2008, p. 148)

---

[1] In a less medicalized form, DI can, and has for a long time also been practiced without medical intervention in a 'do it yourself' fashion (Throsby, 2004, p. 11; Lykke and Bryld, 2006, p. 44).

In becoming 'facts of life', ARTs have helped to denaturalize and diversify hitherto unquestioned binaries, such as nature/culture and biology/sociality as well as sex/procreation, as mentioned above (Inhorn and Birenbaum-Carmeli, 2008, p. 178). In this regard, biotechnical innovations such as reproductive technologies have raised the question of what the 'natural foundations' of life more precisely are and how these differ from 'artificial' life forms (Lemke, 2009). Today, in many ways, we live in a biotechnological culture in which bodies and technologies become increasingly intertwined, reproductive technologies being one example of this development, making it impossible to separate the 'technological/artificial from the organic/natural' (Lykke and Bryld, 2006, pp. 25 and 43). According to Donna Haraway, our bodies have increasingly become technological reconfigured (Haraway, 2004b). These changes include profound shifts in 'the understanding of reproduction as natural, biological processes and of the body as a product of nature' (Lie, 2002, p. 383; Franklin and Lock, 2003, p. 11).

Emphasizing Genetics

It is complicated to grasp the specifics of how the culture/nature relation manifests itself, as several main paradoxes are linked to this distinction. For instance, despite the reconfiguration of 'natural' conceptions, a biogenetic understanding of human nature has gained currency in recent years as a result of medical inventions within the biosciences. An increased focus on 'life itself' both on an individual and political level concerns ways in which we can alter ourselves down to a molecular level. Prenatal diagnosis, stem cell research, genetic testing and IVF technology are just some examples of an amplified concern with biological and genetic questions (Rose, 2001; Franklin, 2008; The Danish Council of Ethics, 2010). This could – paradoxically – imply that 'science has provided another powerful model where human qualities are still based in nature' (Lie, 2002, p. 396). This host of biological issues is joined with another paradox concerning the effects of MAR on family formation – do they for instance promote more inclusive understandings of non-traditional families and 'new families', such as solo mother families?

On the one hand, MAR 'weakens' the influence of the (natural) biological limits to parenthood, since one does not have to rely on the given range of biological possibilities and options in order to become a mother. On the other hand, however, the use of assisted reproduction might enhance the biological interpretation of parenthood since one does not have to rely on social and cultural contracts either. In this regard, it is interesting to ask whether MAR propagates a social, legal, cultural, biological, genetic or technological understanding of parenthood and how these aspects are enacted in everyday practices and form part of the women's self-understandings.[2]

---

[2]I gratefully acknowledge Dr Karen Kastenhofer, researcher at the Institute of Technology Assessment, Austrian Academy of Sciences, for pointing to this duality and its implications for different parenthood understandings.

Choosing to become a solo mother by means of sperm donation entails most often being both a genetic and biological mother to the child (by using one's own eggs and carrying out the pregnancy), as opposed to having become a single adopter for instance.[3] In this case, one might argue that the wish to have a biological child of one's own accentuates a biological understanding of parenthood. At the same time, opting for the use of a donor who will become the biogenetic father but who will probably not enter into any paternal relationship, might indicate that the biological aspect plays a less significant part. Is the wish for an own biological child greater, then, due to the absence of the biogenetic father? Is an identity-release donor preferred for instance, due to the lack of a social father? These questions translate into the broader question of to what extent and in what way single women embarking upon solo motherhood place emphasis on biogenetic and social aspects of kinship, respectively?

Empowering Technologies?

I will return to these paradoxes in subsequent chapters, and continue with another general paradox which has been an area of special concern within the feminist strand of literature theorizing about ARTs. As Charis Thompson (2005, p. 55) writes in *Making Parents,* 'reproductive technologies, and the infertility for which they typically exist to alleviate, pose a paradoxical tension for feminists', since these technologies on the one hand may help defeat involuntary childlessness, which causes many women great distress but on the other hand, they may add to the reproduction and essentializing of gender expectations to reproduction, which can intensify the distress of infertility. The latter precisely constitute the kind of gendered expectations with which feminists have tried to break (Thompson, 2005, p. 55).

Several other issues relate to this paradox and it has long been debated to what extent the possibilities of reproductive technologies should be perceived as liberating for women. Possible consequences and risks have been emphasized, for instance, in terms of women's potential lack of self-determination, aggravation of power inequalities, capitalization and so on (e.g. Brake and Millum, 2012; Adrian, 2006; Franklin, 1993; Ravn and Sørensen, 2013). In general, such feminist theorizing can, very roughly sketched, be placed in the area of tension between technophobia and technophilia and thus between viewing reproductive technologies as a means of oppression or one of empowerment for the women applying the technologies (Adrian, 2006, p. 26). This paradox in terms of empowerment/repression will be explored through the personal narratives of solo mothers in terms of how the technologies influence gender expectations, roles and identities and how the women in this study perceive and approach the use of MAR.

---

[3]An increasing number of single women are also becoming mothers via double donation (both egg and sperm donation) and/or embryo donation (sperm and egg at embryo stage). In this case, the solo mother will not have a genetic link to the child, but she will carry the child and be the gestational mother (Hertz, 2021).

Overview of the Book

Presenting a rich series of biographical narrative interviews with women who have chosen to become solo mothers, the books seeks to explore how life plans, strategies and biographical revisions are transformed, as solo mother families are created in the tension field between the individual and social and between nature and culture. Supplemented by expert interviews, field observations and policy analysis as methods of inquiry, this book aims to show how individual actions, social structures and technological innovations are complexly intertwined and both retain and challenge our existing understandings of – and ways of doing and being family. By treating the subjects of reproductive technology, donor conception and solo motherhood in a holistic fashion the book aims to provide a comprehensive understanding of the interlinkage between personal narratives and social processes and practices.

The biographical narrative interviews were conducted with 22 women during the period of September 2014 to March 2015. At the time of interview, the women differed as to whether they were in treatment, had become pregnant or had conceived a child (an overview of study interviewees is provided in Appendix 1). Biographical narrative research has been applied due to its strengths in eliciting sensitive personal accounts and improve a nuanced understanding of complex meaning-making processes; in reaching in-depth and holistic understandings through broader life stories/transformative experiences and in studying 'lived realities' and narratively explore life plans vs. life changes as well as breaks between real and ideal. Furthermore, the biographical narrative method supports an analytic interlinking of micro and macro processes by attending to the particularities of individual biographies in relation to their sociocultural context (e.g. influence of socio-technical transformations, shifts in reproductive practices) For a detailed overview of methodological aspects, see Appendix 1.

Although reproductive technologies cross borders and national contexts and in many ways can be seen as a global phenomenon, they are still rearticulated and re-contextualized in local settings (Knecht, Klotz and Beck, 2012, pp. 12–13). In many ways, Denmark provides an interesting context. It is a pronatalist welfare state with a rather permissive MAR legislation and free access to health care and reproductive technologies. Denmark has also become 'the fertility hub of Scandinavia' with emerging private fertility clinics and private sperm banking (Kroløkke et al., 2019, p. 1). In this regard, Denmark hosts the world's largest sperm bank, Cryos international, which exports frozen donor sperm worldwide. Likewise, single women from particularly neighbouring European countries travel to Denmark for treatment. Donor-conceived children in Denmark can have donor siblings all over the world and their mothers can – and many do – form online communities with other solo mothers worldwide who has used the same donor (Andreassen, 2018, p. 12). Hence, Danish legislation and policy-making within this area has global implications. In several ways then, solo motherhood in Denmark constitutes a phenomenon that extend beyond a national context and this 'localized' (Jenny, 2013, p. 241) context is also embedded in a broader international setting and within general biocultural transformations. The understanding of 'local' circumstances thus necessitates a broader level of contextualization (i.e. the state of the art from an international perspective, established and emerging field theories) that may function as a broad frame of reference for understanding, more broadly, transformations in science and society in relation to this area of reproduction and family formation.

This book draws on several fields of research. It is informed by sociological conceptions and qualitative research strategies to the studying of empirical phenomena, to social and normative practices and processes as well as to the agency-structure duality in understanding individual behaviour within specific societal contexts. This study is, with its particular focus on ARTs and technoscientific practices, also informed by the broader field of social studies of science and technology and more specifically, feminist science and technology studies (or feminist technoscience studies). The later constitutes in itself a transdisciplinary field of research in drawing from and overlapping and intersecting with cultural studies, feminist studies and science and technology studies (STS) (Lykke, 2008). This book joins and contributes to a small but growing international literature on solo mothers and to the greater field of social and cultural studies on reproductive technologies within feminist literature, within feminist science and technology studies (FSTS), as well as within ethnographic and (medical) anthropological research. Exploring impacts of reproductive technologies through detailed analysis of personal biographical narratives of solo mothers combines interdisciplinary analytical, theoretical and empirical aspects in a way that is novel and particular to this book.

This introductory chapter has framed the objectives of the book and situated the phenomenon of solo motherhood within greater technological, cultural and political contexts. It has presented a number of paradoxes that characterize the developments and expansion of MAR and that revolve around the double feature of both imitating and destabilizing 'natural' forms of procreation and kinship relations. The matter of nature and/or nurture in terms of biogenetic and social aspects of family and kinship formation comes across in the opening statement by Charlotte. Its implications for forming solo mother families will be explored throughout this book. Hence, Chapter 1 examines how MAR has given rise to 'new' family forms. Framed within an international context, the chapter discusses the novelty of such family reconfigurations and the chapter asks where this leave contemporary family life from a sociological point of view? The chapter goes on to examine the solo mother family as a 'new' family constellation and investigates existing studies in this field. Furthermore, through a closer survey into socio-demographic trends and cultural transformations, the chapter discusses a number of contextual particularities that may explain the status of solo motherhood as an emerging family form. Chapter 2 provides a theoretical basis for understanding the phenomenon of solo motherhood by way of assisted reproduction. The chapter explores three different theoretical perspectives, which individually and collectively inform and deepen the empirical analysis of the book. Overall, the book argues throughout that we need to transgress – and not dissolve – nature/culture binaries and seek instead to explore how social and biogenetic aspects interact with, and substantiate, each other in reproducing and disrupting established practices of reproduction and kinship making. This argument draws from and adds to the theoretical scholarship of (1) feminist theoretical concepts related to the sociocultural implications of reproductive technologies, (2) theoretical concepts within the field of new critical kinship theory and theories on 'doing family', and (3) narrative and social identity theory. The combination of STS oriented theory on kinship transformation and processual identity theory allows for new insights into the complexities of how solo mothers 'do' family and identify themselves as solo mothers in a continuing negotiation of normalizing and naturalizing the choice to create life as a single parent. Chapter 3 sheds light on the political and discursive context of legislating access to assisted reproduction in Denmark. It outlines the MAR policy landscape and compares it to European policy changes within the area. The chapter then delves into a detailed analysis of the policy transformations that has taken place in Denmark regarding access to MAR. The chapter theorizes reproduction as an area of tension between the private and political and argues that an emerging new governing rationality can be identified that reflects new biopolitical forms of regulation, risks and subject constructions in line with the concept of ethopolitics. Chapter 4 continues with the lived effects of the legislation on equal access to MAR and explores the relations between the personal and the social and between the private and political from the individual point of view through personal narratives of contemplating solo motherhood. It shows how the attainment of equal rights and benefits have added to the women's notions of solo motherhood being a viable, moral and acceptable route to motherhood. The chapter examines how solo mothers motivate their decision to embark upon solo motherhood and how their choice can be understood biographically and within the specific sociocultural and legal context in which the decision is made. Chapter 5 seeks to provide a first account of how single women manage and navigate the process of undergoing fertility treatment. It shows how understandings of 'natural processes' are subject to change over the course of treatment and how boundaries and distinctions shift and transform throughout. It is discussed how the process of fertility treatment influences the lifeplanning/biographical revisions made by the women. Furthermore, the chapter describes the emotional and physical aspects and strains of undergoing treatment and shows how they reinforce one another. The interdependence of bodily and discursive processes (nature-culture) is analytically expanded and related to how bodies are managed and 'biological responsibility' enacted, for instance in terms of treatment decisions, life style changes and in the adherence to the time-tabled nature of treatment. Chapter 6 shows how solo mothers define and create family and focuses on how the interplay between biogenetic and social aspects are negotiated and redefined in relation to the desire to have a child of one's own, and its implications for attachment, motherhood and identity issues. It furthermore details how the women negotiate kinship as both an imagined and lived practice and how family and network relations are actually established. In interlinking biographical particularities with the meaning of an 'own' child, five distinct strategies are invoked by the women to motivate and legitimate the choice of donor conception as a route to motherhood. Chapter 7 explores how the women in the study choose and relate to the donor as well as relate to potential donor siblings. As established by existing research, the genetic donation poses a paradoxical tension: while the donation itself is embedded within existing kinship systems, donors will often not take an active part in the child's upbringing, at least until the child reaches adulthood. In the wake of genetic inheritance becoming more significant and greater donor openness being established through cross-country policy measures, comes the question of whether donors are conceptualized as kin or as non-kin? The distinct Danish two-way donor model that allows donors and recipients to decide the degree of openness surrounding the donation is discussed, and the women's different rationales for choosing a donor are compared. The chapter shows that clear kinship boundaries are difficult to manage, and it illustrates the often complex and challenging discipline of fitting, and situating, the donor and donor siblings within ordinary kinship categories. The final Chapter 8 concludes the book by summarizing and interlinking key findings, and revisits to the main paradoxes presented in the introduction. By doing so, it charts and clarifies the complex entanglements of individual, technological, legal and sociocultural aspects emphasized when life as a solo mother is planned, revised, created and lived.

Chapter 1

Creating Life as a Solo Mother: An Emerging Phenomenon?

The proliferation of medically assisted reproduction (MAR), such as in vitro fertilization (IVF), has influenced and facilitated the rise of 'new' kinship practices and family formations. Yet, to what extent and in which ways our existing ideas about family and kinship conceptualizations have been challenged and revised, do not seem to yield straightforward answers. By examining how MAR has given rise to 'new' family forms as well as discussing the novelty of such family reconfigurations by examining the 'traditional' historical aspect of the nuclear family model, this chapter seeks to contribute to the ongoing question of how biological and social aspects inform and define kinship and family formation (Edwards, 2009).

The chapter goes on to examine the solo mother family as a 'new' family constellation and, through a closer survey into socio-demographic trends and cultural transformations, points to a number of contextual particularities that may explain the status of solo motherhood. For instance, by looking at changes in reproductive practises, fertility patterns, cultural circumstances, the meaning of motherhood etc., can we identify developments and conditions, which support the prevalence of single mothers by choice as an emerging family type? The case study, on which the book is based, is situated in a Danish context, and specific socio-cultural factors – such as supportive welfare structures and free access to fertility treatment – are taken into consideration but contextualized within a broader international setting and within more general bio-cultural transformations.

In outline and as a frame of reference for the findings in this book, the chapter concludes by assembling what we already know about this growing group of women and the well-being of their donor-conceived children.

1.1 MAR and the Formation of 'New' Families

By separating human procreation from sexual relations, reproductive technologies have facilitated a change in how families can be (and are) formed and structured, effectively blurring familiar categories associated with parenthood, paternity and maternity. For instance, it is possible for a child to have up to five parents: An egg donor (the genetic mother), a sperm donor (the genetic father), a

Lived Realities of Solo Motherhood, Donor Conception
and Medically Assisted Reproduction, 15–34
Copyright © 2021 Tine Ravn
Published under exclusive licence by Emerald Publishing Limited
doi:10.1108/978-1-83909-115-520211002

gestational (surrogate) mother who hosts the pregnancy ('birth mother'), and the two social parents whom the child recognizes as mother and father (Golombok, 2015, p. 16; Melhuus, 2012). These 'new families' created by means of assisted reproductive technologies and potentially through donated eggs, sperm, embryos or surrogacy began to emerge at the end of the twentieth century. New families include for instance families headed by solo mothers or solo fathers, lesbian mother families, gay father families, co-parents that are not romantically involved and donor-conceived families at where a two-parent heterosexual couple for instance become parents through egg or sperm donation, which imply that the child will not have a genetic link to one of its parents. The 'new families' are seen as more distinct from the 'traditional' family form than 'nontraditional' families formed by cohabiting parents or by single parents or stepparents at where families are often recomposed due to divorce or separation (Golombok, 2015, p. 16; Golombok, 2020, see also introduction). Families that are donor-conceived – such as the solo mother families in this book – face a number of novel considerations about what constitute kin for them. How are they to relate to the donor, to potential donor siblings and to their families? The forcing of such relationships and the potential for new forms of kinship and relatedness add to the question of how the meaning and establishment of family and kinship evolve over time.

While there is little doubt that reproductive technologies have challenged our normative understandings of what constitutes and defines a family – despite ongoing discussion of the extent to which 'normative categories' have been trans-gressed or merely reinforced – it is also important to emphasize that changes in family demographics and transformations regarding family practices also occurred before the birth of Louise Brown. For instance, in Europe and North America, families were increasingly 'recomposed' due to divorces and remarriages, an increasing number of children were born out-of-wedlock, making unmarried cou-ples and single parents more mainstream and less stigmatized. Same-sex partners, too, saw an increased level of acknowledgment (Carsten, 2004; Franklin and McKinnon, 2001; Levine, 2008; Melhuus, 2012; Mortelmans et al., 2016). I will return to these social changes later, but for now simply stress the point that several transformations and shifts – among these, the responses to MAR – have challenged the hegemonic status of the nuclear conventional family and helped stress kin relations as more fluid in nature. While they may still appear 'congealed', this does not mean they are 'preexisting' entities, as Franklin and McKinnon accentuate (Franklin and McKinnon, 2001, p. 13; Levine, 2008). To rephrase this, kinship is both part of nature and culture, found in a position between both something 'given' and something 'made', despite more essentialist assumptions, which base kin relations on a set of 'natural facts' (Carsten, 2004, pp. 9 and 167).

1.1.1 The (Non)-'traditional' Nuclear Family Formation

In this aspect, the nuclear family based on romantic (heterosexual) love, marriage and co-habitation (also termed 'heterorelationality'), including the genetically related children, still remains naturalized and an idealized family form for many. Since the nineteenth century, and in Europe and North America in particular, 'natural kin' primarily connotes biological relations in establishing kin, which is a contrast to family practices found on other continents where 'blood or marital ties' are not necessarily decisive for forming social relations (Budgeon and Roseneil, 2004, p. 129; Cutas and Chan, 2012, p. 7; Christiansen, 2007; Levine, 2008, p. 378; Lock and Nguyen, 2010, p. 265; Ottosen, 2005, p. 19).

> The idealizing ideas that surround the small nuclear family today, as well as its assumed historical authenticity, turn out to be difficult to locate in reality, both presently and historically speaking.
>
> –Christiansen (2007, p. 8)

Thus, 'the "traditional family" is not all that traditional' (Nicholson, 1997, p. 27) and some of the basic characteristics associated with this traditional family form were simply enabled by social changes taking place during the eighteenth and nineteenth century in Western Europe and North America. In a Danish context, the nuclear family structure gained currency among the working class segment during the industrialization and urbanization of the late nineteenth century, partly due to the fact that urban apartments often only allowed for two residing adults, which often meant having to leave one's own parents behind in the countryside. Notwithstanding the nuclear structure, the living, working and family conditions of these late nineteenth century urban families, significantly differed from today's standards (Christiansen, 2007).

Leaping ahead, the nuclear family structure presumably seen as 'traditional', emerged and expanded after the economic boom that occurred post World War II alongside the rise of a growing middle class. However, flanking the 1950s family model, other factors such as increasing divorce rates, as mentioned above, gave rise to the formation of new types of families (Nicholson, 1997, pp. 27–28). The 'second demographic transition' (SDT) characterized by increasing divorce rates, postponement of child births and more non-married couples choosing co-habitation, occurred from the 1970s onwards, and were rendered possible by a growing number of women entering the paid labour force from the 1960s, the prevalence of modern contraception and changes in family values, among other features. Overall, the transition refers to demographic and interconnected changes and trends related to family construction, fertility and partnership conduct that are linked to broader macro structural, cultural, technological and economic changes such as modernization, secularization and individualization (Ottosen, 2005, pp. 18–19; Sobotka, 2008, p. 172). In addition to the value oriented and ideational underpinnings of the second demographic transition that emphasize growing individual autonomy and anti-authoritarian values, Mortelmans et al. point to two additional theoretical frameworks that may help account for the developments witnessed in Europe and beyond from the 1960s and 1970s and onwards (2016). The 'new home economics' framework advanced by Gary Becker draws attention to the opportunity costs related to marriage and parenthood due to the growing paid labour participation by women; increased economic independence prompts emancipation and provides new options for women such as being able to leave an unhappy marriage. Third, the 'incomplete revolution' framework by Esping-Andersen seeks to explain developments and variation across countries in family dynamics and social inequality from the late twentieth century by an increasing gender-equality equilibrium, at where the shifting roles, behaviour and preferences of women in relation to education, domestic work, career and family life in particular drive shifts in demography and family dynamics (Esping-Andersen, 2009; Mortelmans et al., 2016, p. 2).

The historical transformations make it clear that the 'traditional' family is neither a natural, nor a universal phenomenon – an observation that renders the distinction between 'traditional' and 'alternative' family constructions questionable. Furthermore, the content of the 'traditional' is also subject to change – the nuclear family we know today does not resemble the 1950s version much, with its stay-at-home mothers and constricted, standardized timing of marriage and parenting, for instance (Nicholson, 1997).

1.1.2 The Decline of the Family?

Today, real-life practices reflect that families come in all shapes and sizes, including single parents, same-sex partners, rainbow families, 'electively or circumstantially childless families', blended families and donor-conceived families. These changes in family demographics, along with the proliferation of assisted reproduction, have raised questions as to what the grounds of parenthood are, what good parenting requires and what the permissibility of MAR should be. Furthermore, debate regarding the proliferation of assisted reproduction has also revolved around whether access to these technologies could possibly threaten the very foundation of the nuclear family structure, since reproductive technologies have expanded precisely on the basis of their potential to create new types of family forms (Brake and Millum, 2012; Cutas and Chan, 2012, pp. 1–2; Norup, 2006, p. 69). Thus, the increase of 'new' families made possible by reproductive technology has fuelled the debate about what a family 'ought to be' in epistemological and moral terms (Silva and Smart, 1998, p. 1) and sharpened the more general rhetoric regarding the decline of the family; a rhetoric which has influenced the public and political debate in many countries, and to which distinctions to growing divorce rates, delinquency, single parent households etc. have been drawn (Carsten, 2004, p. 181; Silva and Smart, 1998, p. 1).

From a sociological perspective, the decline of the family supposition in a western context has been related to increased rationalization and individualization, which has rendered the conventional nuclear family structure ever more unstable and divorced from its former, traditional functions. However, despite social changes, the family as a social institution and a 'social organization principle' (Ottosen, 2005, p. 17) remains resilient and the answer to what comes after the family is according to Beck-Gernsheim still, 'the family!'. However, as a 'post-familial family', in new multiple guises, forms and variations, seen in the light of changing social structures and normative contexts, but also within a range of newly accessible options (Beck-Gernsheim, 2002, p. 6; Budgeon and Roseneil, 2004; Ottosen, 2005; Schultz-Jørgensen and Christensen, 2011).

Despite individualization processes – or perhaps due to them – the family unit, whatever form it may take, then remains, and still offers a central frame of reference for personal anchorage, identity construction, social fulfilment, and solidarity – possibly because it represents to many, an anchor in an 'uncertain society, which has been stripped of its traditions and exposed to all sorts of risks' (Beck-Gernsheim, 2002, p. 8) and possibly because work pressures, performance and ever growing demands of efficiency and effectivity also force us to prioritize our social relations. Hence, the increased possibility to design individual life trajectories has not superseded the family as an important institution. Rather the family has adapted well to societal transformations. In addition to the explanations suggested above, indicators of this continued force is found to be 'the persistent high value attached to family and children and the overwhelming positive attitude towards parenthood' (Sobotka, 2008, p. 209).

When the family holds such a significant position in the construction of individual biographies, accordingly it is held to high standards 'of which new social meanings are continuously ascribed to the family as an institution in order for it to function optimally' (Christiansen, 2007, p. 18; Ottosen, 2005, p. 20). Presumably, the pressures of these heightened and continuous standards put a strain on family relations, which are in themselves, already brittle. As mentioned by way of the second democratic transition, and despite variation within and across countries, an increase in both divorce rates and co-habitation has been observed 'throughout much of the industrialized world' (Perelli-Harris et al., 2017, p. 303; Kennedy and Ruggles, 2014; Sobotka and Toulemon, 2008).

1.1.2.1 Family Demography

In a Danish context, 46% of all marriages in 2018 ended in a divorce (compared to 44% in 2010, 2000, and 1990). The divorce frequency has up until 2011 been relatively high on the percentage rate, but have at the same time been stabilized (Schultz-Jørgensen and Christensen, 2011, p. 32; Statistics Denmark, 2020a). From 2012, the divorce frequency rose to its highest rate of 54% in 2014 and decreased again in the following years. Interestingly, from 2018 to 2019 the frequency dropped by 30% from 46% to 35%. It is yet to be seen whether this movement can be accounted for by a change in legislation in 2019 that introduced a three-month reflection period for couples with shared children before the realization of a divorce (Statistics Denmark, 2020b).

The number of people who have not married has increased and people are also getting married later in life. Hence, 66% of all 30-year-olds were married in 1980 compared to 28% in 2016. Still, 2017 figures show that 75% of all couples living together are married. On the other hand, the figures also show that around one third of the adult population live as single (Statistics Denmark, 2017). The figures paint a varicoloured picture of the modern family and in this respect, it is interesting to note that the central authority on Danish statistics operates with 37 distinct family structures. To take this one step further, does this then imply the end of the nuclear family as we know it? Figures from 2019 show that 73% of all children below the age of 18 live with both their parents. By comparison, only 16% of 16-year-olds did not live with both their parents in 1980. 'Couple families' constitute 45% of all family types in 2020 compared to 49% in 1990. 43% of the couple families have children living at home. Whereas the couple family has decreased, the single family (of which 11% has children living at home) has increased from 50% (1990) to 55%. In the UK and USA, the number of families headed by single parents has also risen from 10% in the 1970s to around 30% (Brejnholt, 2013, p. 5; Golombok, 2015, p. 16; Statistics Denmark, 2020c). Furthermore, within the last decade, the number of rainbow families have more than doubled and 27% of same-sex partners have children living at home (Statistics Denmark, 2019).

The statistical trends reveal both variation and continuity in family life, and whereas the two-parent model still seems to dominate existing family practices and is by no means rendered obsolete, 'this organization no longer defines so exclusively what it is like to live in a family, or what a family *is*' (Silva and Smart, 1998, p. 4). It is possible then, that increased family diversity, enabled among other factors by means of reproductive technology, may have helped highlight the 'doing' of family life (emphasis on the 'made' rather than the 'given') while stressing how individuals themselves ascribe meaning to, and define family practices and kin relations, rather than merely following a pre-given order of things. Of course, the 'doing' of family still takes place within different normative contexts, a point being that such contexts undergo transformations as well, notwithstanding the often inert processes of such changes.

1.1.2.2 Variation in Sociocultural Practices
Despite the transforming effects of MAR, assisted fertility practices are also seen to adapt to existing sociocultural practices. To explicate such variations and their implications for kinship relations, examples from other parts of the world prove illustrative. For instance, third party conception is not allowed in Egypt due to perceptions regarding adultery, risk of incest amongst offspring and the great importance attached to genealogical relations. Instead, male infertility is treated with a procedure of intracytoplasmic sperm injection (ICSI), where sperm is injected directly into the egg (Carsten, 2004; Franklin and McKinnon, 2001; Kooli, 2019; Levine, 2008; Silva and Smart, 1998).

The concerns of adultery and the risks of incest among offspring also entered into former rabbinic debates about donor insemination in Israel; the outcome and rationales involved in these, however, were quite different from those of Egypt. Furthermore, in these debates, two other circumstances also played a part; that masturbation is forbidden for orthodox Jewish men and that only matrilineal descent determine the Jewish identity of the child. According to interpretations of Jewish law, non-Jewish donor sperm was then seen by the rabbinate to be the best choice in cases where donor insemination was needed. Adulterous relations only pertain to Jews, which essentially meant that the use of non-Jewish sperm did not qualify as adultery to the same extent as, for example, a case in which a child was born as the result of an actual (Jewish) adulterous relation. Additionally, since non-Jewish paternity is not recognized in Jewish law, the infertile Jewish husband can establish paternity through his intention to do so. In fact, children born to separate mothers but using the same non-Jewish donor-sperm are not perceived as related. The strong 'matrilineal ethos of Judaism' (Bock, 2000, p. 79) focuses attention on reproduction and supportive fertility treatment and reimbursement policies, and in so doing has also supported the growing trend among single, Israeli Jewish women to form solo mother families through donor insemination. Furthermore, children born to Jewish single mothers by choice do not suffer from any of 'the stigma associated with Euro-American notions of bastardy' (Levine, 2008, p. 283; Birenbaum-Carmeli, 2016; Carsten, 2004).

These examples demonstrate that biological, social and genetic factors are intertwined in very complex ways, as are the public – private spheres (Carsten, 2004; Levine, 2008; Franklin, 2013b). The examples also illustrate a variety in the ways in which kinship and family relations can be created and negotiated, and that the specifics are dependent on sociocultural contexts, interlinking micro and macro processes.

1.2 Socio-demographic Trends and Cultural Transformations: The Significance of Children and Motherhood

As much as the 'status' of family life today in all its various shapes and sizes constitutes an important contextual piece in the greater framework puzzle of understanding solo motherhood, so too do the more general socio- and bio-demographic trends in terms of reproductive practice. Therefore, to understand the 'choice' of establishing solo mother families, it is equally important to understand the cultural significance attached to children and motherhood/parenthood today.

With MAR, human reproduction and sexual relations have increasingly been separated. A similar separation was also initiated with increased birth control from the 1960s onwards, a development which was fuelled by the persistence of the women's movement; improved contraceptive devices such as the introduction of the contraceptive pill (in the 1960s) and the introduction of abortion on demand (in 1973 in Denmark), both of which increasingly enabled women to control their own fertility and likewise plan the timing of family formation. Other socio-demographic factors which have contributed to the delaying of childbirth have been increased and prolonged education, increased workforce participation, financial insecurity and lack of partner, among others (Norup, 2006, p. 51; Knudsen, 2009; Knudsen, 2014, p. 171; Rosenbeck, 1995, p. 21).

1.2.1 Age, Fertility and Family Policies

With regard to delayed childbearing, the average age for being a first-time mother was 29.5 in 2019 in Denmark. The general average of 31 years in 2019 for women given birth has particularly increased since 1970 when the average age was 26.7, compared to around 23 in the early 1960s. Despite fertility postponement, the completed fertility in Denmark has increased from a trough of 1.38 in 1983 to 1.70 in 2019. The rate was also 1.70 in 2014, at where France and Ireland with 2.0 had the highest European fertility rate and Portugal had the lowest fertility rate with 1.2 (Statistics Denmark, 2020d; Statistics Denmark, 2017; Knudsen, 2009). An increased proportion of women postpone having children until their late thirties and early forties with rising infertility as a consequence. Still, research suggests that even though childbirth is postponed, the intended number of children planned can still be reached. However, as Sobotka et al. (2008, p. 80) also point out; 'younger cohorts of Danish women may find it increasingly difficult to reach their desired family size as they face rising infertility due to fertility postponement'. Hence, looking at the past 50 years, the number of children born per woman has decreased – a tendency which has been termed 'lowest low fertility' (Knudsen, 2009, p. 13) – and an increasing proportion have remained childless. For instance, in 1991 the share of woman that remained childless at the age of 50 was 8.2 compared to 12.9 in 2009 and 11.9 in 2018. Nevertheless, even though the Danish fertility rate is lower than the required population replacement level, compared to other European countries, the Danish fertility rate remains relatively high (Knudsen, 2009; Sobotka et al., 2008, p. 80; Statistics Denmark, 2017).

Increased opportunities to plan *not* to have a child by means of contraceptives, for instance, have also led to a belief that it is possible to choose to have a child *when* planned for it (Knudsen, 2009). However, returning to bio-demographic factors, the delay of childbearing – termed 'ageing of fertility' – 'increases the proportion of couples having fertility problems, increases the risk of becoming a fertility patient, and increases the risk of remaining childless or having fewer children than desired' (Schmidt, 2010, p. 145). As Schmidt furthermore emphasizes, reduced fecundity due to increased age cannot be fully negated by use of assisted reproductive technologies. Along with environmental and lifestyle factors then, which can negatively affect men and women's fertility, a range of socio-demographic and bio-demographic factors can help explain developments in fertility practices. In the same vein, despite increased opportunities to plan family formation at an agency level, many factors cannot be controlled individually. For instance, such a factor could be enhancement of existing family policies. For example, improved conditions for student families, additional flexible leave arrangements and day care could underpin earlier family formations while also supporting life-work balance at large (Knudsen, 2009; Schmidt, 2010). Still;

> The welfare state system, characterized by important features such as access to leave schemes for both parents, sufficient access to day care facilities and equality between spouses, is in general considered to provide a proper framework for childbearing and child rearing.
>
> –Schmidt (2010, p. 146)

Increased equality between men and women is expressed both de jure and de facto, leaving women independent and able to provide for themselves and their children after a possible divorce, due to their education and work force participation. Thus, such conditions also enable single women to form solo mother families (Knudsen, 2009; Frederiksen, 2010).

Furthermore, in line with the arguments above, enhancement of family-friendly policies and 'a more gender-egalitarian welfare state' are increasingly seen as supporting of higher fertility rates (Ellingsæter et al., 2013, p. 6; Esping-Andersen, 2009, p. 14). Still, welfare system facilitation of reproductive practices must be seen in the context of access to assisted reproductive technologies. As assisted reproduction remains a 'stratified possibility' in many countries so too do supporting welfare policies;

> The implementation of social changes (including good maternity leave policies, provision of high-quality, inexpensive childcare and other forms of maternal support) that would facilitate the realization of these procreative desires more universally remains strikingly limited in the United States, Britain and many other Western Countries.
>
> –McNeil (2007, p. 83)

In many ways, Danish family policies have found a 'proper framework for childbearing and child rearing' (Schmidt, 2010, p. 146) as mentioned above. Combined with equal access to MAR and supportive reimbursement policies – which is a unique constellation also in comparison with other Scandinavian countries – it is a presumption in this book that such welfare policies constitute a supportive factor in understanding the prevalence of Danish single mothers by choice as an emerging family type, while also making the formation of solo mother families a less 'stratified possibility' (Schmidt, expert interview; Salomon et al., 2015, see Chapter 4).

Cultural changes have taken place and it seems as though different family formations have received greater social acceptance, including the single parent family. Acceptances of the latter have been explained by an actual increase in divorces and likewise a greater proportion of the population living in single parent families (Schultz-Jørgensen and Christensen, 2011). Possibly, this growing acceptance will also come to include single mothers by choice, even though they are perhaps more exposed to the need to justify their choice of intentionally acting as the sole parent, straying away from the most common two-parent route to family formation which – regardless of their current family situation – is originally taken by divorced single women. As a result, according to Bock (2000, pp. 65–66), they 'do not need to justify their parental status'.

1.2.2 The Significance of Children and Motherhood

Today, despite the fact that an increasing number of women remain either voluntarily or involuntarily childless, 'motherhood is constituted as compulsory, normal and natural for women, for their adult identities and personal development...' (Woollett and Boyle, 2000, p. 309). Motherhood and parenthood have been democratized and if we consider the greater historical timespan, a greater proportion of women experience motherhood within a generation today than was the case a 100 years ago. For instance, 25% of all women born in 1907/08 never became mothers; possibly because their financial situations never allowed for it (Norup, 2006, pp. 51–52; Rosenbeck, 1995, pp. 18–19; Schmidt, 2006, p. 390).

> At the individual level, reproduction is a result of the most intimate human behavior. At the same time, the decision to have children is influenced by economic, social and cultural forces, as reflected in the systematic variation in fertility levels across countries, social groups and over time.
>
> –Ellingsæter et al. (2013, p. 4)

Following such historical variations, the meaning of motherhood and fatherhood is transformative as well. For instance, in a Western context, maternity has increasingly been seen as inextricably linked with motherhood, in this way also interlinking 'giving birth and giving nurture' (Gillis, 1996, p. 153) while supporting the accepted cultural norm that having one's own (biological) child is significant (Rosenbeck, 1995). But why is having children influenced by such strong normative notions, naturalizing and essentializing motherhood as a consequence? The 'social meaning of children' (Ellingsæter et al., 2013, p. 5) can be seen in parallel with the continuing significance attached to the family unit in terms of creating a central frame of reference for identity construction and social fulfilment, among others, as earlier described. In this regard, children tie the family unit together (Tjørnhøj-Thomsen, 2003, p. 67). Thus, recalling the quotation by Hertz, stating that solo mothers' 'decisions to become a mother reflect the broader mandates of American culture that tie motherhood to womanhood, parenthood to adulthood' (2006, p. 19), correspondingly emphasizes that motherhood is also in a broader Western context 'regarded as an inevitable part of a woman's normal life course' (Sevón, 2005, p. 462) and forms an important part in the forging of identity.

The cultural and social significance of children also becomes evident through the accounts of those who are involuntarily childless. As Tjørnhøj-Thomsen (2003) shows, the meaning of children is highly entangled with feelings of 'being right' in terms of being a member of society in a proper fashion, being part of history by carrying on the family lineage as well as belonging to various kinds of social communities to which children enable access. Hence, having children 'provide(s) authenticity, a sense of belonging and identity in an uncertain modern world' (2003, p. 79).

Furthermore, others have observed that a normalization of motherhood not only relates to becoming a mother or not, but that dominant cultural narratives also define the criteria for '"good" mothering and a "reasonable" female life course' in terms of timing and quality assessments (Sevón, 2005, p. 461; Woollett and Boyle, 2000). How these and other sociocultural narratives and expectations regarding parenthood and motherhood influence the women in this study will be explored in later chapters. Paradoxically, if the above-mentioned cultural discourses prevail, and if neither remaining single nor being a single mother form part of predominating cultural narratives, how are they then to define and negotiate family and kin? Furthermore, how does the use of assisted reproductive technologies enter into such negotiation and normalization processes?

1.3 Single Mothers by Choice as 'New' Families

The literature on single mothers by choice represents a growing body of work; still, the extent of studies carried out remain relatively limited in number and in scope. The majority of studies that have been conducted have primarily taken place in the US and UK, and in the UK predominantly within the Centre for Family Research at The University of Cambridge. The following sections will broadly review recent literature which centres on single mothers by choice. Against this backdrop, it will explore existing knowledge around questions such as: Are there specific character-istics which are shared by this particular group of solo mothers? What motivates single women by choice to pursue solo motherhood and what are their main con-siderations during the decision-making process? Furthermore, much debate on whether or not single (and lesbian) women should be able to access assisted repro-duction, have been focused on the question of the well-being of the prospective child in terms of the 'need for a father'. In the UK, this was a prevailing topic with regard to the 2008 Human Fertilisation and Embryology Act (Gamble, 2009) and likewise in the Danish debate on this matter as detailed in Chapter 2. Existing knowledge on how children thrive in solo mother families will be delineated in terms of the effects of this family form on parenting and development issues.

1.3.1 Socio-demographic Characteristics

Single mothers by choice (SMCs) or solo mothers are women who intentionally choose to conceive a child and act as the sole parent and who differ from mothers who have become single-after-the-fact, due to factors such as divorce, separation or the death of a partner (Graham and Braverman, 2012, p. 189; Golombok, 2015, p. 115). Furthermore, in the literature, single mothers by choice are often described as a distinct group of solo mothers who are financially independent, well-educated, middle to upper-class women in their late thirties and forties with well paid jobs and supportive social networks of family and friends (Bock, 2000; Grill, 2005; Jadva et al., 2009a; Malmquist et al., 2019; Mannis, 1999). The coining of the term 'single mothers by choice' by Jane Mattes in 1982 aimed to describe a group of responsible, mature and empowered women who *chose* to enter motherhood (Graham and Braverman, 2012). At the same time, 'the label itself serves to separate this population from other single mothers, those who allegedly are the "real" problem'. By this, Bock (2000) refers to the pejorative terminology which has frequently been associated with single mothers historically;

> The terms single mother and welfare-dependent have consequently come to be highly intertwined, adding to the stereotype of the

> single mother as lazy and unmotivated, sexually irresponsible, and young (...). In many ways, the 'new' single mothers inherit the stigma of their poorer younger sisters.
>
> –Bock (2000, p. 63)

Due to social, political and cultural developments, among other factors, having a child out of marriage does not imply the same stigma as was earlier the case (Bock, 2000; Weinraub et al., 2002; Mazor, 2004; Scott et al., 2019). However, despite an increasing number of single parents over the last 20–30 years, single parents remain exposed to criticism, in some cases to such a degree that single parenthood came to be seen as 'a kind of social pathology' and catalyst for major social problems (Weinraub et al., 2002, p. 109; Murray and Golombok, 2005a). Such views were fuelled by early research on fatherless families, which found negative effects in terms of emotional, cognitive and behavioural problems in children raised in single mother families. However, these studies focused mainly on children which – following the separation or divorce of their parents – grew up with their mothers only. Subsequent studies have shown that such negative outcomes can be ascribed to factors such as socio-economic disadvantages, children experiencing parental conflicts, maternal depression and a lack of social support – thus factors relating to the social context rather than paternal absence as such. Since children of single mothers by choice are not exposed to risks associated with parental divorce, the negative effects on children as described above may not concern children in solo mother families, where the mothers' level of psychological well-being has been found not to differ from a married DI mother's (Graham and Braverman, 2012; Golombok, 2015; Golombok, 2013; Grill, 2005; Murray and Golombok, 2005a). In fact, as will be further detailed below, children raised by single mothers by choice seem to be thriving very well.

While single mothers by choice have separated themselves from other groups of single mothers to avoid criticism and legitimize their choice of parenting alone (Bock, 2000), others have suggested the broadening of the definition of single mothers by choice;

> Many women – poor as well as rich – find themselves pregnant and choose to remain single and rear their child without the presence of a male partner. Could they too not be considered single mothers by choice?
>
> –Weinraub et al. (2002, p. 126)

The active choice to become a single parent defines this group of women and this possibly constitutes a more significant factor than the specific route to motherhood. In this light, this growing group of women worldwide is probably more diverse in terms of socio-economic characteristics than originally described in the literature (see for instance studies by Jones, 2007 and Hertz, 2002, which include working-class SMCs). However, if the route to solo motherhood implies accessing MAR, the 'choice' of pursuing solo motherhood remains a largely 'stratified possibility' in many countries, available only to those who can afford fertility treatment at private clinics. In the UK, funding of treatment cycles is prioritized differently in different areas of the country, resulting in unequal access to treatment and skewed waiting times (Graham, 2014; Shenfield et al., 2010). Single women – with or without a medical infertility diagnosis – are not likely to receive fertility treatment funded by the National Health Service (NHS). For instance, only one woman embarking upon solo motherhood through MAR received funded treatment by the NHS out of 23 single women participating in a study by Graham (2014; Graham and Braverman, 2012). In the US, a similar inequity of access is observed by Charis Thompson (2005, p. 26),

> On a nationwide scale, the inequities that stem from disparities in access to treatment and in quality of treatment have proven to be more resistant to change than any of the inequities that were specific to reproductive technologies, such as judgments about who is worthy to be a parent.

In Denmark, where fertility treatment in public clinics is free of charge, it is likely that the diminishment of inequity of access has an impact on the demographic composition of the single women pursuing solo motherhood via MAR. In a Danish multicentre survey spanning 300 women, a comparison of 184 single women and 127 cohabiting women undergoing fertility treatment with donor semen found no 'significant differences [...] regarding sociodemographic characteristics, previous long-term relationships, previous pregnancies or attitudes towards motherhood..' (Salomon et al., 2015, p. 473). The main difference between the two groups was a difference in age. With an average age of 36.1, the single women were in general 3.5 years older when treatment was commenced than the group of cohabiting women. Findings have shown that higher levels of reimbursement have a positive influence on national birth rates and the number of assisted reproductive technology (ART) cycles performed. In 2011, a 50% co-payment scheme on assisted reproduction in the public health care system was introduced in Denmark. Based on the one year, the scheme was in effect, it resulted in a 30% reduction in treatments in public clinics and it is estimated that this represents the birth of approximately 700 fewer children as a direct consequence of the reimbursement policy (ESHRE, 2012; Erb, expert interview p. 37; for a complete review see Schmidt and Ziebe, 2013).

1.3.2 Motivating Driving Forces and Life Situations

Not surprisingly, the one main motivating force for embarking upon solo motherhood is the wish for a child, a wish often expressed as an 'overwhelming drive for motherhood' and a 'desire to nurture' (Graham, 2012, p. 101; Mannis, 1999, p. 124; Golombok, 2015). As Rosanna Hertz states in her book *Single by chance, mothers by choice* (2006, p. 19), which comprises a study of 65 SMCs,

> These women's decisions to become a mother reflect the broader mandates of American culture that tie motherhood to womanhood,

parenthood to adulthood. Their decision is akin to that made by their partnered heterosexual peers, although it is not sheltered by social norms.

It is of course important to remember that all single mothers by choice (like everyone else) are carrying their various personal histories and that the decision to pursue solo motherhood is based on a variety of reasons, rationales, life situations, etc. I will return to the cultural and social element encompassed in the quotation above; however the quotation also emphasizes that the reasons for solo mothers to contemplate solo motherhood do not fundamentally differ from others' reasons for entering parenthood. In this regard, research suggests that most single mothers by choice do not intentionally want to deselect a partner and/ or father for their prospective child but that this 'choice' of opting for solo motherhood must be understood as a 'plan b' when faced with limited possibilities to find a suitable partner within the biological time-frame of being able to conceive a child. A general finding furthermore suggests that most single mothers by choice would have preferred to have a child within a relationship. With this being a limited option, motherhood is prioritized first while a potential partner may come subsequently (Bock, 2000; Golombok, 2015; Golombok, 2020; Graham, 2012; Grill, 2005; Frederiksen, 2010; Frederiksen et al., 2011; Hanson, 2001; Mannis, 1999; Murray and Golombok, 2005a; Volgsten and Schmidt, 2019). In contrast to this, one finding from a large scale survey conducted by Jadva et al. including 291 women, reported that around one third of the women without a current partner had chosen to stay single (2009a, p. 182).

Echoing other findings, this did not imply that these women did not find the presence of male role models to be of importance to their children or that they experienced difficulties with forming intimate long-term relations as is sometimes presumed. Instead, in this particular study, the majority of women had previously been in long-term relationships but for a number of reasons (the relationship or timing was not right, the partner did not want children etc.), the relationships did not provide the desired foundation for family formation. Furthermore, several studies find that the ideal of the nuclear family is not abandoned but merely reworked and postponed (Bock, 2000; Graham, 2012; Hertz, 2006; Jadva et al., 2009a; Mannis, 1999; Murray and Golombok, 2005a). Based on an interview study with 26 SMCs, Bock (2000, p. 70) makes the following observation:

> In some sense they appear to be 'unwilling warriors' who, on the one hand, stress the importance of having the option of single motherhood, yet, on the other hand, cling to hegemonic fantasies of normative family structures.

Bock furthermore found that remaining close to the nuclear family ideal, and the norms and values inherent within the 'normative social order', formed part of the process of legitimizing and normalizing their decision to depart from the traditional family formation trajectory (Bock, 2000, p. 70). In addition, Mannis (1999) reported that the women in her small-scale interview study to some extent seemed to want to reproduce their own and often more traditional family experiences, while also being influenced by social and cultural changes in relation to 'workplace opportunities', 'changing and emerging social institutions' and 'feminist ideas' (Mannis, 1999, p. 124).

1.3.3 Contemplating Solo Motherhood – A Branch of Complex Decision-Making

That the decision-making process is complex, deliberate, well-planned and based on a number of careful considerations is well documented within the existing literature. In the above-mentioned study by Bock, it was found that four key attributes were crucial to the decision to legitimize the choice of entering into solo motherhood: age (increasing), responsibility, emotional maturity and financial means (2000). Likewise, Leiblum et al. reported secure employment, the biological-clock-related concern of 'time running out', processing and settlement of parenthood concerns, as well as social support as main decision impactors (1995). Furthermore, many women make practical arrangements in advance to secure the best possible conditions for the child; this includes saving money, moving to a new neighbourhood, making career changes and securing social network support to assist with childcare (Jadva et al., 2009a; Graham and Braverman, 2012, p. 200; Frederiksen, 2010).

> The intentional and planned manner of their pursuit of parenthood, the support of others, as well as the love and time, they felt they could give a child became incorporated into their ideals for family life.
>
> –Graham (2012, p. 107)

Graham further emphasizes that the 'potential child seems to be at the forefront of decision-making' and much thought is given to how their decision to pursue solo motherhood will influence the well-being of the child. Friends, family and health professionals, among others, have also often been consulted in the decision-making process. One main issue in this regard has been referred to as 'the daddy issue' and thus concerns how the child will react to not having a 'designated' or 'known father'. However, the conviction that the women will be able to create loving and caring homes for their children and provide for them financially and emotionally, 'outweigh' the concern regarding the absence of a known father. A male influence is still valued significantly by most women and many make sure that male role models within their family and social networks are available (Bock, 2000, p. 76; Golombok, 2015; Graham, 2012; Graham and Braverman, 2012; Jadva et al., 2009a; Jones, 2007; Leiblum et al., 1995, p. 16).

1.3.3.1 Routes to Solo Motherhood and Choice of Donor

Single women can pursue single motherhood in a number of ways and the choice of method varies according to preferences, moral beliefs and the options available. Research however suggests that a majority of women choose fertility treatment with donor sperm at fertility clinics (Jadva et al., 2009a; Graham, 2014; Golombok, 2020). With regard to the latter, an interesting issue regarding the women's concerns about the absence of a designated father relate to the women's choice of donor. This is not just a de facto matter of choosing between an anonymous or known donor; the decision enters into the complex decision-making process outlined above, and becomes entangled with matters of moral convictions, perceptions of kinship and relatedness, complex understandings of the meanings and implications ascribed to the donor, as well as statutory demands (Graham, 2014; Landau et al., 2008; Hertz, 2002).

With regard to the latter, identity-release sperm donation has been required in the UK since 2005, whereas it in Denmark – whether to use anonymous or non-anonymous sperm donation – has been optional since October 1, 2012. Previously, medical professionals were only allowed to use sperm from anonymous donors for treatment, whereas private midwifery clinics could offer insemination with either open or anonymous donor sperm (Law 602 of June 18, 2012). However, not much research has been conducted on the rationales and motivations of single mothers by choice regarding the choice of donor, herein the significance of the donor vis-à-vis the welfare and identity-formation of the child. The recent study by Graham found that the majority of the women in her study preferred identity-release sperm donation because they felt the child had a 'right to know' and should be able to contact the biological father at some point. This conviction stems from the belief that knowledge of a child's genetic origin plays an important role in the child's identity formation. The five women in the study who chose anonymous sperm donation, primarily due to the necessity of seeking less expensive fertility treatment abroad, were concerned about the anonymity of the donors, partly because the children would grow up in a UK setting where access to donor information has become statutory and thus their children might also expect to be able to access information about their donor (Graham, 2014).

Chapter 7 explores how the 2012 Danish donor amendment has influenced the women in this particular study, in relation to how they position themselves in the matter of donor type, the significance they place on the identity of the donor and the importance of knowledge of genetic origin in relation to identity formation. These themes relate to the importance of biogenetic ties and the greater paradox of whether and in what sense medical assisted reproduction propagates a genetic, biological or social understanding of parenthood. The afore-mentioned study by Graham suggests that great importance was attached by the women to 'having a child of their own' and being both biologically and genetically related to the child (the three women in the study who used double donation with both donor eggs and sperm, were still biologically related to their children by virtue of gestating and giving birth to their child).

Interestingly, while some women stressed the genetic element of carrying on the family lineage, for the majority of women, the connotation of a child of their own was seen 'to be as much about being pregnant, gestating a child and giving birth to it, as about passing on their genes'. In the same manner, the unknown element of not knowing the donor – as a real person with distinctive features – proved a much larger issue than the question of genetic heritage (Graham, 2014, p. 5). Although the meanings and perceptions of social, genetic and biological parenthood are clearly intertwined in complex ways, the desire for a child of their own also partly relates to the wish to 'normalise their route to motherhood and to retain some elements of traditional procreation and the nuclear family they had imagined for themselves'. This is also reflected in a tendency for the women to personify the donor to some extent based on the information released (Graham, 2014, p. 4).

This alignment to, and reaffirmation of the nuclear family ideal, also resembles other findings, and as described above, this kind of normalization as it occurs in the choice of single motherhood is closely connected to the strategy of legitimizing the choice itself. In the study by Hertz, 'women contextualize the donors that allowed them to become mothers through acknowledging the social ways that blood kinship creates families' (Hertz, 2002, p. 1). Information about the biological father and donor entered into the construction of an 'imagined father' figure that both helped affirm the child's identity and make it seem akin to its peers (Hertz, 2002, p. 1; March, 2008). Although the 'conception story' changes when technology is involved (Thørnhøj-Thomsen, 1998, p. 23), it was refashioned so as to be aligned to more traditional conception stories. Furthermore, as Hertz describes,

> The storytelling is in part genetic and in part social. The importance of genetics is a contradictory arena from a medical perspective, particularly with regard to how much weight to give genetics in shaping lives over nurture. But from a purely social perspective, genetics is both an idea and a road map of identity.
> –Hertz (2002, p. 3)

The biological father and donor hold a distinct role as an 'imagined father' in the solo mother family and in the study, the women sustain a boundary between social and genetic kinship, maintaining that only one man can be the father of the child. Interestingly, Hertz holds that this boundary is maintained due to a wish for a partner – and social father – to emerge and adopt the child (Hertz, 2002, p. 26). While this may be taken in support of more traditional kinship structures, it is also a way of rendering the biological aspect less important. Is donor knowledge then more important in solo mother families due to the absence of a social second parent (Graham, 2014, p. 15), and because less emphasis is placed on the genetic and biological elements as such? Furthermore, how is this related to the normalizing processes mentioned above, aligning to more traditional family patterns? (See Chapter 6 for 7 for an exploration of these questions.)

1.3.4 The Well-Being of Children in Solo Mother Families

Concerns about the psychological well-being of children raised in solo mother families have in particular been an issue due to early research on fatherless families; nonetheless, no evidence suggests that these negative outcomes apply for children raised by single mothers by choice.

Yet, at the same time, it has been indicated that children in solo mother families might be exposed to an 'increased psychological risk' due to the lack of a designated father figure and the fact that the mother's route to parenthood combines the two more or less controversial ventures of donor insemination and single motherhood (Golombok, 2012, p. 64). However, existing studies available on the matter find that these children function very well and conclude that there is nothing to indicate that they experience any disadvantages by being raised in solo mother families. A longitudinal UK study, comparing DI solo mother families to married DI families (27 solo mother DI families and 50 married DI families in the first study and 21 versus 46 in the follow-up study) found no negative effects with regard to the quality of the parent-child relationship and the psychological well-being of the mothers at year one and two of the child. In fact, the latter follow-up study found that the children in solo mother families showed 'fewer emotional and behavioural difficulties' than in the comparison group of children in married DI families, although all were functioning well (Murray and Golombok, 2005a, 2005b, p. 242). Similarly, a US-based cross-sectional study found that donor-conceived children at age seven were well adjusted and well-functioning. The study included 80 families, which varied according to family structures, e.g. such as number of parents and parents' sexual orientation. Another significant finding showed that behavioural problems and child adjustment were related to family processes such as parental stress and parental conflict, rather than the nature of the particular family structure (Chan et al., 1998). Another study detailing 62 Israeli DI solo mother families found that the children's socio-emotional development could be placed within a normal range (Weissenberg et al., 2007).

In terms of long-term effects, a longitudinal study detailing the socio-emotional developments of children, as well as the quality of parenthood in mother-headed families (including both single, heterosexual mothers and families headed by lesbian mothers), found no negative effects regarding either the quality of the mother-child relationship or the well-being of the child as a result of growing up without a resident father from infancy. Findings from the children at age 6 (Golombok et al., 1997), 12 (MacCallum and Golombok, 2004) and 18 (Golombok and Badger, 2010) were thus comparable to those from the two-parent heterosexual families. Interestingly, the authors report in the third follow-up study (at year 18) that:

> Where differences were identified between family types, these pointed to more positive family relationships and greater psychological well-being among young adults raised in female-headed homes.
>
> –Golombok and Badger (2010, p. 150)

For instance, the young adults from mother-headed homes 'showed lower levels of anxiety, depression, hostility and problematic alcohol use' than the young adults in the two-parent heterosexual families as well revealing greater self-esteem (Golombok and Badger, 2010, p. 156). The study furthermore challenges theories stating that the lack of a father causes a change in children's gender identity, understood in terms of boys being less masculine and girls less feminine than children reared in families with a father present. The study further disproves theories claiming that parents influence the development of children's sexual identity, (e.g. that children in lesbian families also grow up to be lesbian or gay). The study shows that by year 12, the boys in mother-headed families were no less masculine-oriented in their gender role behaviour than their peers despite the fact that they also showed more 'feminine characteristics' which is explained by these boys being supported in showing 'sensitive and caring attitudes'. Regarding sexual identity, at year 18 all identified themselves as heterosexual except for one young woman, who identified as bi-sexual (Golombok and Badger, 2010; Mac-Callum and Golombok, 2004, p. 1416).

Another recent follow-up study comparing 51 solo mother families with a match comparison group of 52 two-parent families with a donor-conceived child at the average age of 5½ found no differences between the family types in regard to child adjustment and parenting quality. As to the latter, lower mother-child conflict was found in the solo mother families. In both family types, parenting stress and financial strains were linked to higher levels of children's' adjustment problems (Golombok et al., 2016). In the second phase of the study, 41 of the solo mothers and 37 of the partnered women took part when the children were around the age of 8–10. Maternal mental health, relationship between mother and child and child adjustment were investigated through standardized interviews, questionnaire and observation. While the first study did not show a decrease in psychological well-being due to the children not knowing their biological father, children first begin to understand biological inheritance in middle childhood. The second phase of the study investigated whether children transitioning into this phase in childhood and being born to solo mothers were at risk for psychological difficulties. As in the first phase of the study, overall, children in both types of families were functioning equally well. The study concludes that 'even when donor-conceived children of single mothers reach the age at which they understand the significance of not having a father, they are no more likely to show adjustment difficulties than children who grow up with a father' (Golombok et al., 2020, p. 8).

In general, research on solo mother families as well as other types of families suggests that the quality of family relations constitutes a decisive factor for children's psychological well-being rather than how families are created and structured (Murray and Golombok, 2005a; Golombok et al., 2020).

This chapter has attempted to make out the contours of the sociocultural landscape and explore existing knowledge on solo motherhood to illustrate the complex entanglements of individual and sociocultural influences for this field of research. A rising number of single women choose to embark upon solo motherhood (see introduction for details). Overall, this chapter explores and argues that the following factors can be highlighted as relevant contextual particulars to expound on the emergence of solo mother families:

- Greater family diversity and greater acceptance of a variety of family practises
- A general trend of delaying childbirth while accordingly reducing the time span for reproduction
- Existing supportive welfare structures
- Sociocultural significance attached to having children

Evidently, such factors must be seen in interplay with the proliferation and refinement of assisted reproductive technologies, and the introduction of legislative changes.

Chapter 2

Theorizing Reproductive Technologies: Negotiating Nature and Nurture in Kinship and Identity Making

This chapter brings together three different theoretical perspectives that individually and collectively provide a framework for understanding the phenomenon of solo motherhood by way of medically assisted reproduction. This book argues throughout that we need to transgress – and not dissolve – nature/culture binaries and seek instead to explore how social and biogenetic aspects interact with, and substantiate, each other in reproducing and disrupting established practices of reproduction and kinship making. This argument draws from and adds to the theoretical scholarship explored and mapped in this chapter: (1) feminist theoretical concepts related to the sociocultural implications of reproductive technologies, (2) theoretical concepts within the field of new critical kinship theory and theories on 'doing family', and (3) narrative and social identity theory. The combination of STS oriented theory on kinship transformation, sociological theorizing about families and processual identity theory allows for new insights into the complexities of how solo mothers 'do' family, engage with reproductive technologies and identify themselves as solo mothers.

> Theory is meant to orient, to provide the roughest sketch for travel.
>
> –Haraway (2004a, p. 63)

Theories are always situated within specific historical and cultural contexts. They are 'siting devices' according to Donna Haraway, and 'mappings' through which to explore particular research landscapes. As Haraway asserts in 'The Promises of Monsters', theory is 'a mapping exercise and travelogue through mindscapes and landscapes of what may count as nature in certain local/global struggles' (Haraway, 2004a, p. 63). To Haraway, theory functions as a tool to disrupt the distinction between social constructions (culture/discourse) and natural objects (nature/materiality).

Haraway challenges and transgresses established identity categorizations and dichotomies such as culture/nature, which may appear to us as natural, universal and normalized, in order to explore complex and ambiguous ways of being and

Lived Realities of Solo Motherhood, Donor Conception
and Medically Assisted Reproduction, 35–54
Copyright © 2021 Tine Ravn
Published under exclusive licence by Emerald Publishing Limited
doi:10.1108/978-1-83909-115-520211004

the possibility for new and different stories (Haraway, 2004b). To Haraway, both discursive and material processes are closely intertwined in the formation of organisms. The body, for instance, is created in a complex interplay between dominating discursive practices and technoscientific interventions but it is also a pre-discursive fact, a material matter beyond our control (Haraway, 2004a). Haraway addresses the fusion between bodies and technology and its influence on our understandings of gender and identity (Haraway, 2004b). Accordingly, in this book, the use of assisted reproductive technologies serves as precisely such a fusion, one which disrupts the nature/culture distinction to alter our understandings both of how we are made and of 'natural' categories such as family and kin (Thompson, 2005). The understanding of such fusions and their implications for the nature/culture distinction – and more specifically for our understanding of identity, gender, family and kin – runs as a thematic thread through this chapter.

Taken together, the three main theoretical mappings 'provide the roughest sketch for travel' in navigating the empirical landscape of solo motherhood, in a changing context of medically assisted reproduction (MAR) and new family and kinship practices. By bringing three different but interrelated theoretical mappings into the dialogue, this work aims to explore intersections between them, in order to sketch out new roads for theoretical travel. Fundamentally, the different mappings function as analytical and thematic divisions, and are represented by interdisciplinary thinkers who come from and transgress different fields of research in science and technology studies (STS), kinship and family studies and gender theory.

2.1 Theorizing Reproductive Technologies: Perspectives and Positionings

Since the 1970s, the use and impacts of assisted reproduction have been increasingly important to feminist theory and debate. Questions such as whether reproductive technologies are to be viewed mainly as a means for improving women's reproductive choices or whether they should be seen as reinforcing patriarchal and medical control over women's bodies, have been discussed at length (Adrian, 2006; Courduriés and Herbrand, 2014). Over the years, much has been written on this topic, leading to an impressive body of work which can be largely characterized by a certain 'technological ambivalence' (Franklin, 2013a, p. 185). As such, the multifaceted meaning of 'choice' and the broad variety of technological techniques (e.g. from prenatal screening to IVF procedures) complicate the adoption of a clear-cut for-or-against approach to reproductive technologies. Despite this ambivalence, the feminist approaches to reproductive technology – especially from the 1970s until the early 1990s – range from those of the technophobic to those of the technophile. The early hope that assisted reproduction, and the future development of an artificial womb, could free women from the biological boundaries of reproduction, famously asserted by Sulamith Firestone in *The Dialectic of Sex* from 1970, was replaced by much more critical voices from other radical feminists, who rejected the technologies

altogether (Adrian, 2006; Courduriés and Herbrand, 2014). In general however –
although there were outliers – most feminists' responses to assisted reproduction
throughout the 1980s were in keeping with 'the more technophobic, antieugenicist
and antipatriarchal sentiments of radical feminism' (Thompson, 2005, p. 57).

Sarah Franklin and Charis Thompson argue that the preoccupation with
reproductive technology within feminist theory can be attributed to the technologies condensing of 'so many of the social, economic, and political stratifications
that affect women's lives and selves, while also foregrounding the tension between
accommodation to the status quo and resistance' (Franklin, 2013a, p. 187;
Thompson, 2005, p. 56). The theoretical matter of reproductive technologies is
also one that intertwines with matters of gender, sexuality, kinship, reproduction,
power, stratification and other topics central to feminist theory. Thompson also
asserts that specific writings and approaches to reproductive technologies, roughly
divided into two phases, to some extent correspond with second-wave and third-
wave (poststructuralist) feminism. Broadly speaking, the first phase of theorizing,
which emerged after the birth of Louise Brown in 1983, was characterized by
technophobic reactions as noted above.

The new reproductive technologies, many radical feminist feared, could prove
to simply provide a new means for men to exert control, not just over women's
sexualities but also their reproduction. In this light, reproductive technologies
were seen as routes to the objectification of women and the reduction of female
bodies to sites of medical experimentation and treatment, with a low actual
success rate in terms of the alleviation of involuntary childlessness. Moreover, the
eugenic aspects of sex selection, along with the commercialization of women's
bodies through surrogacy and egg donation, were highly problematized. Such
criticisms used the matter of reproductive technology to raise feminist issues of
gender, class and race stratification and discrimination, which were key areas of
concern for second-wave feminists (Thompson, 2005; Adrian, 2006). Many of the
issues related to 'stratified reproduction' (i.e. reinforcement of social and structural inequalities in the global 'reproductive bioeconomy' (Waldby and Cooper,
2008, p. 58)) continue to be central in feminists studies of reproductive technology
today.

The views held by the radical feminists outlined a clear distinction between
nature and culture and likewise between what was seen as natural and artificial;
the new technologies were inherently seen as repressive, and natural childbirths
were called for. Men and women were positioned as essentially different, by
maintaining that the technological developments would prove advantageous to
men and not to women (Adrian, 2006). The critical argument – that reproductive
technology would serve to maintain and reaffirm extant sex/gender divisions (and
a nature/culture distinction), and that such technology took all women as one
unified subject and neglected differences among women – is a more general
critique that pertains to second-wave feminism (see Butler, 1999). Such criticism,
as raised by third-wave or poststructuralist feminists, is reflected in the second
phase of theorizing reproductive technology: Throughout the 1990s, the issue of
stratification remained central but the technophobic and patriarchal approach to
assisted reproduction was replaced by a more nuanced and ambivalent approach.

The techniques and success rates of assisted reproduction improved; feminist researchers within the natural sciences started to approach the techniques from a technical, yet still critical, point of view, and feminist writers increasingly focused their attention on the issue of infertility.

Women's and men's various lived experiences of infertility, their motivations for undertaking assisted reproduction and the physical and emotional experiences of treatment became the subject of a number of empirical studies that theorized the relation between the personal and political, between agency and social structures and increasingly also between the discursive and the material (see e.g. Adrian, 2006; Becker, 2000; Franklin, 1997; Thompson, 2005; Tjørnhøj-Thomsen, 1999; Trosby, 2004). According to Thompson, the second phase framed the issue of infertility within a 'transnational politics of reproduction' (2005, p. 74) and despite the great variety of studies across themes and research fields, feminist researchers adopted a much more social constructivist approach that marked a break with essentialized understandings of gender and a clear distinction between nature and culture; instead, the practical negotiations and implications of this distinction were – and continue to be – explored empirically (Adrian, 2006).

2.1.1 Donna Haraway and Charis Thompson: Theorizing Material-Discursive Processes

While the social-constructivist approaches merely focused on the individuals applying the technologies, taking its point of departure in human experiences or on how materialization processes are made possible through discursive norms and regulations (see e.g. Butler, 1999), a growing number of researchers, located within the science and technology (STS) tradition among others, started to address the materiality of reproductive technologies and of bodies and cells. The material may act in surprising ways, and it may potentially influence processes of change, for instance in terms of existing practices and sociocultural norms (Adrian, 2014). In addressing the 'agency of bodily matter' (Lykke, 2010, p. 120), Haraway underlines that the body is not to be seen as either passive or static, but as a living fact beyond our complete control. Haraway recapitulates her position in the following way:

> I am neither a naturalist, nor a social constructivist. Neither-nor. This is not social constructionism, and it is not technoscientific, or biological determinism. It is not nature. It is not culture. It is truly about a serious historical effort to get elsewhere.
>
> –Haraway (2004b, p. 330)

Haraway uses the term 'material-semiotic actor' to refer to the ontological duality embedded in the processes of becoming (i.e. the creation of organisms) and which includes the intertwinement and interdependence of both techno-cultural discourse and biological materiality (2004a, p. 67). Haraway's figuration of the 'apparatus of bodily production' (2004a, p. 67) is closely connected to the transgression of the material/discursive distinction. As do Foucault and Butler, Haraway sees the body as an object of scientific knowledge production that is shaped by dominant and institutionalized discursive practices. Yet Haraway transgresses this constructionist positioning by emphasizing two additional points; as captured by the 'agency of bodily matter' mentioned earlier, bodily materials will always be a living fact beyond our control, and bodies are moreover always created in interaction with various techno-scientific interventions (Haraway, 2004a; Lykke, 2010).

For instance, while technological interventions within the field of reproductive technology have rendered possible a separation between sexual relations and procreation in destabilizing biological facts, a woman's biological age remains a key determinant for the success rate of fertility treatment. For instance, for women over the age of 40 the success rate is significantly lower than for women below the age of 40 (ESHRE, 2016). Female biological age serves here as one illustration of biological materiality that can be influenced by medical interventions but remains nonetheless beyond our full control. At the same time, the age limit for starting treatment – 40 years for women in the public health sector and 46 years in the private one – is also a sociocultural construct and regulated by law. Other countries such as Spain and the UK, for instance, do not operate with the same age criteria. This small example illustrates the need to contextualize and 'situate' studies of technology, as Haraway emphasizes (Adrian, 2014) whilst also serving to illustrate how matters related to biology, discursive practices, technology and the personal interweave. On the personal level, biological age as a 'biological fact' influences the biographical facts, playing for instance a significant role in life-planning (and biographical revisions) in the process of contemplating motherhood.

The ground-breaking ethnographic study by Charis Thompson – most comprehensively presented in *Making Parents* (2005) – broadly details the 'interaction between patients and the medical technology' (2005, p. 179) at infertility clinics. Encompassed by the concept of 'ontological choreography', Thompson shows how the process of making individuals into parents by means of reproductive technology depends on a 'dynamic coordination of the technical, scientific, kinship, gender, emotional, legal, political and financial aspects of ART clinics' (2005, p. 8). Processes related to the personal, the technological and the political are all fused together in complex ways and are closely intertwined with processes of naturalization and normalization. Inspired by the STS tradition and in particular Haraway's situated approach to technology and knowledge objects in general, Thompson integrates a focus on materiality (e.g. bodily and technological processes) with a focus on human agency and the different subject positions adopted by potential parents during treatment. For the patient undergoing treatment, a number of ontological transformations take place during the course of treatment. The stories told and the experiences emphasized are likely to change throughout the different phases of treatment depending on the individual's personal situation and the success/failure of treatment cycles, among many other factors. Consequently, the individual patients undergo a process which also influences their self-understanding and identity construction (Adrian, 2006; Markussen and Gad, 2007; Thompson, 2005). Furthermore, for many, the process of undergoing fertility treatment can be characterized as an 'emotional rollercoaster' (Thompson, 2005,

p. 93) as a result of the many emotional ups and downs and the level of stress related to undergoing treatment. Experiences of success and failure during treatment can trigger alternating states of hope and despair; the reactions to hormone treatments can be emotional and physically trying, and the more practical aspects of juggling weekly treatment appointments with a full-time job can be stressful (Thompson, 2005, p. 93).

Thompson argues that 'we cannot presuppose an ontology of the unified subject because a coherent self-narrative requires ontological heterogeneity' (Thompson, 2005, p. 182). As in the narrative approach (see Appendix 1), contradictions in a told narrative are not to be perceived as problematic but indicate subjective and contextual changes in the course of treatment. For instance, the rationalizations for why a treatment results in a pregnancy or why it is unsuccessful in reaching this goal, may come across differently in the narrative regarding the way in which aspects of the technical, natural and social are emphasized. As Thompson exemplifies, one unsuccessful cycle may be described as objectifying and alienating, whereas an identical cycle resulting in pregnancy might be described very differently. Hence, 'the context of the self has moved and the nature of the account helps to fix the identity of the patient at the time she is speaking' (Cussins, 1996, p. 590; Thompson, 2005, p. 203). The notion of 'ontological choreography' also expresses the key idea that technological objectification and individual agency are not antithetical to one another. Consequently, Thompson dismisses the more technophobic strands within feminist studies that perceive reproductive technologies as objectifying women per se in oppressing agency and self-hood. She also shows that objectification does not automatically translate into states of alienation. Rather,

> The women's objectification involves her active participation, and is managed by herself as crucially as it is by the practitioners, procedures and instruments. The trails of activity wrought in the treatment setting are not only not incompatible with objectification, but they sometimes require periods of objectification.
>
> –Cussins ((later Thompson), 1996, p. 580)

Sometimes the woman is seen as a patient with a complete medical and personal story, at other times she is objectified according to a number of standardized practices, or perceived merely through body parts (e.g. ultrasound screen pictures of ovaries and follicles). According to Thompson, these ontological changes involve an interlinkage between agency and objectification that are coordinated or choreographed to maintain a sense of being a 'whole person' (Cussins, 1996, p. 600; Thompson, 2005, p. 182).

The concept of 'ontological choreography' and, more broadly, Thompson's dynamic and contextual approach to studying patient-technology interaction acts as a framework in this book for interpreting the experience, meaning and use of reproductive technology. In Chapter 5, I explore whether the women in this research for instance change their perceptions of medically assisted reproduction during the process of treatment; whether a process of normalizing and naturalizing different forms of assisted reproduction (e.g. IVF and egg donation) take place and whether they adopt different subject positions during treatment influencing their self-understanding.

In 'Making Parents', Thompson explores how patients manage and choreograph the biogenetic facts of reproduction with social categories of kinship. By means of assisted reproduction and third party genetic donations (from sperm and egg donors and surrogates), new kinship relations are created. This does not mean that the more familiar and traditional kinship categorizations are dismissed, nor that they form the sole basis for doing kinship. Rather, through the concept of 'strategic naturalization', Thompson shows how patients claim kin by strategically emphasizing some elements of biological reproduction and excluding or downplaying other elements. This complex choreography between natural and cultural aspects of kinship reveals not a clear nature/culture distinction but rather that the two are 'used to generate and substantiate each other in specific cases' (2005, p. 147). With this concept in mind, the next section seeks to continue and expand the theoretical framework for discussing the implications of medically assisted reproduction on contemporary kinship and family formation.

2.2 New Kinship Studies and Theories on 'Doing Family'

How are we to understand contemporary analytical and theoretical conceptions of kinship and family? The question does not yield unequivocal answers within or across the academic traditions that have sought to answer it. Such concepts are, naturally, in a state of flux: they develop in line with changes in society, and in general, and are subject to continuous change in the actual ways kinship and families are formed. Within the field of anthropology, kinship studies remain vital despite periods of transformation and reinvention. Driven forward by the rise in reproductive technologies and in the growth of new family forms – partly made possible by biotechnical developments – the 1990s saw the emergence of the notion of 'new kinship studies' which remains central in research today (Edwards, 2009; Franklin, 2013b; Franklin and McKinnon, 2001). This section presents an outline of the new kinship studies as well as sociological theories related to the concept of 'doing family', with the aim of framing these theoretical approaches within broader empirical and theoretical developments, not only to situate them as 'siting devices' but likewise, to frame the fields of research wherein this book is situated.

2.2.1 The Emergence of New Kinship Studies

Empirically, the new kinship studies are shaped by developments in reproductive technologies and family demographics, as noted above. The work of anthropologist David Schneider (1918–1995) to reconfigure kinship theory in terms of biological vis-à-vis social aspects, serve as a notable theoretical source for revitalizations within the field of the new kinship studies. Schneider's critique of extant approaches to kinship occurred as a part of a larger, general trend in anthropology's thematic and conceptual shift 'from function to meaning' (Carsten, 2004, p. 18) and heralded a parting with the Euro-American structural and functionalist view of kinship as a social structure and the nuclear family as a main societal organizing principle (see e.g. Radcliffe-Brown and Malinowski), and a divergence from the structuralist approach represented by Lévi-Strauss. Lévi-Strauss was concerned with the universal rules which he thought to structure human kinship relations, such as marriage relations (men exchanged women) and incest taboos (to secure marriage across groups) (Carsten, 2004, see this source for a review; Franklin and McKinnon, 2001). The departure from such approaches was also a shift towards the more 'self-critical and reflexive approaches' which came to characterize anthropology in the 1970s and 1980s (Franklin and McKinnon, 2001, p. 3).

Schneider's influential critique of earlier approaches to kinship is a two-fold one; first, it problematizes the Western kinship model for treating sexual reproduction as a natural fact which defines kinship relations across cultures. To Schneider, kinship cannot be pre-defined in such terms – rather, its definition should always be a matter of empirical study within cultures. Second, Schneider rejected the approach of treating kinship as a separate and distinct analytical domain and asserted that to argue from, or for, pre-defined kinship categories which were separate from other domains such as politics, economics and religion for instance, would be to fail to capture the diverse cultural practices of kinship (McKinnon, 2015) that do exist. In this light, Schneider held that to view kinship as merely grounded on the biological facts of sexual reproduction would amount to hold a mere tautology, since

> The notion of a 'base in nature' creates a self-justifying and untestable definition of kinship: 'kinship' as a sociocultural phenomenon is, in the first instance, defined as entailing those 'natural' or 'biological' facts which it is at the same time said to be 'rooted in' or 'based on'. The phenomena which are shown by analysis to be related are already related by definition.
> –Schneider (1984 in Franklin and McKinnon, 2001, p. 2)

Schneider problematized the nature-culture distinction and hence the a-priori distinction between biological and social aspects of kinship; his critique of the biological foundation of kinship focused primarily on the ethnocentric aspect of applying Euro-American understandings of kinship as a universal model. He did not draw attention to variations within a culture, nor did he criticize the naturalization of categories such as gender, which were inherent to the 'biological' based kinship model. The problematization of 'natural facts' as a basis for kinship constructions has since been taken up by multiple researchers; Feminist researchers, for example, have critiqued the fixed understandings of 'natural' gender categories as a basis for reproduction and kinship constructions (Carsten, 2004; Franklin and McKinnon, 2001). In the first major critique of these 'natural facts', Yanagisako and Collier argued that instead of applying 'naturalized differences' as taken for granted concepts, the 'cultural assumptions' inherent to our understandings of kinship as cultural and historical practices, need themselves to be subject to study, if we are to understand both kinship conceptualizations and actual kinship practices (Franklin and McKinnon, 2001, p. 4).

In this regard, the new kinship studies were driven by two main 'imperatives' according to Edwards (2009). First, efforts were made among anthropologists to highlight the social aspects of kinship and to show how social connections were established through feeding and caring for instance. At the same time, this was a departure from the view of biology as a particularly privileged or distinguished marker of kinship, and an effort to avoid kinship definitions that might reinforce biological determinism. Second, in line with developments in assisted reproduction technologies (ARTs), anthropologists increasingly focused on issues of science and technology, and with inspiration from STS studies, a focus on biology in terms of 'the culturally constructed body' was brought back onto the research agenda. The gendered and social aspect of gametes and hormones, for instance, became topics of theoretical and sociological enquiry which focused on bodies in relation to biomedicine. According to Edwards, the studies, however, maintained a constructivist research approach and tended to maintain a distinction between 'the biological' and the 'social' (2009, pp. 3–4).

With the rise of new reproductive technologies, the question of nature and culture remained central. The seminal work of Marilyn Strathern, and in particular her books *After Nature* and *Reproducing the Future* (both 1992), have had a strong influence on the new kinship studies. Strathern, looking at English culture in the late-twentieth-century, argued that nature no longer could 'be considered as the grounding for culture, or as simply there to be revealed or discovered. It is as least partly "produced" through technological intervention...' (Strathern in Carsten, 2004, pp. 21–22). In this view, kinship is to be seen as a hybrid between nature and culture, an entity which interconnects both 'domains'; it is reproduction as 'enterprised-up', to use Strathern's term. As aspects of social parenthood are increasingly recognized by law, Strathern says, there follows the growing difficulty of believing nature to be something 'independent of social intervention' (Carsten, 2000, p. 10). Strathern believed her position to have implications not only for kinship and kinship studies but indeed for the very prospect of the attainment of knowledge in general: If nature itself is subject to transformation, then knowledge is not only something out there for us to simply 'discover' – rather, knowledge (like kinship) must be to a certain degree made and created in a manner that is at least partially divorced from natural factors (Carsten, 2000; Carsten, 2004; Franklin and McKinnon, 2001).

As Carsten states in her book *After Kinship*, it 'seems impossible to move between kinship and gender without passing through bodies' and she suggests the integration of biological processes in the study of kinship (2004, p. 27). As opposed to maintaining a distinction between biological and social aspects, as in the earlier studies mentioned above, the 'new' kinship studies seem to focus increasingly on the 'oscillation' between the two domains (Edwards, 2009, p. 14), with one exemplary issue being the way in which reproductive technologies serve to destabilize the biological and 'natural' foundation for the way kinship is established; or as Mason puts it: 'As biology itself transforms, we cannot any longer see it expressing the "given" facts of kinship' (2008, pp. 31–32). This destabilization or denaturalization of previous established kinship models, in favour of a broader and more dynamic view of relatedness, is central and it also involves new understandings of bodily substances such as blood, genes and other biogenetic substances (Mason, 2008, pp. 31–32; McKinnon, 2015, p. 564).

> Not only within biological science but also within biological bodies, it has become more difficult to determine what it means to speak in 'strictly' biological terms. What I am describing here as both the 'new biologies' (by which I mean the material-semiotic practices of the contemporary biological sciences) and 'new biologicals' (by which I refer to new entities such as cryopreserved human embryos, cloned transgenic animals, genetically modified seeds, and patented gene sequences) can be said to defamiliarize the very nature of what it is to do biology or be biological.
>
> –Franklin (2001, p. 303)

Franklin argues that the aspect of 'biology' continues to matter but that the definition of biology is no longer by any means 'self-evident' and that consequently, any analysis will require 'careful contextualization' in order not to either overstate or undermine innovations related to the biological (Franklin, 2001, pp. 304 and 317). In *Biological Relatives*, Franklin explores the paradoxical workings of IVF in what she terms 'the age of biology'. By this she refers to the transformations taking place in the relationship between biology and technology, which consequently reflects the contingency of biology (Franklin, 2013a, p. 8). The focus on biological contingency and dismissal of fixed and reductionist models is in contrast to the emergence of the field of genetics and 'the gene's-eye-view' of the world which emphasizes nature over nurture (Rose, 1997, p. 6).

In the wake of the Human Genome Project, advances in DNA, genetic testing, gene therapy and so forth; genetic thinking has become increasingly prominent in scientific and public discourses.[1] Furthermore, in contemporary Western societies, the view of genetics and genes as an explanatory mechanism for individuals' personal traits, behaviours, health conditions, sexual orientation and talent has found its way into our daily life practices and language to such an extent that we may by now refer to it as a kind of 'geneticization of society' (Nordqvist and Smart, 2014, pp. 144ff; Nordqvist, 2017; Hertz and Nelson, 2019, p. 5). As Donna Haraway has also pointed out, we now live in an age in which – when mental health issues are detected for instance – our 'first explanation for such things is a genetic explanation' (Haraway, 2000, p. 149; see also e.g. Rose, 2001, 1997).

---

[1] The aim of The Human Genome Project (HGP) was 'to sequence and map all of the genes – together known as the genome'. This large international project was launched in 1990 and officially closed in 2003 (National Human Genome Research Institute, 2016).

Certain biologists and geneticists have themselves sought to challenge the reductionist aspect of geneticization (Edwards, 2009). For instance, in *Lifelines – life beyond the gene*, biologist Steven Rose argues that 'genes and environment are dialectically interdependent throughout any individual's lifeline' (1997, p. 133). Siddhartha Mukherjee argues that we cannot 'speak about "nature" or "nurture" in absolutes or abstracts' but that the development of certain features is contingent upon the context and the single feature. Human attributes are often 'the results of collaborations between genes, environments, and chance' (2016, pp. 480–481).

While it is argued that the geneticization thesis has lost some of its explanatory power as it has failed to account for the complexity of biology and fails to 'tell the whole story of human life and relatedness', it has still influenced our everyday understandings of kinship and inheritance and served to reinforce the importance of genetic connections (Nordqvist and Smart, 2014, pp. 155ff). Featherstone et al. argue that while reproductive technologies blur the distinction between 'biological facts of conception and the social categories of kinship', genetics (e.g. genetic testing) serves to reinforce 'conventional categories of reproduction and related-ness' (cited from Edwards, 2009, pp. 11–12). The new kinship studies have theoretically and empirically addressed how such developments impact under-standings of kinship and the paradoxical ways in which kinship emerge as both something 'given' and something 'made' (Carsten, 2004, p. 9).

On the one hand, reproductive technologies – in obscuring the relation between 'biological facts of conception and the social categories of kinship' – have challenged existing normative ideas about family constructions and kinship conceptualizations (Edwards, 2009, p. 11; Levine, 2008; Melhuus, 2012). On the other hand, others have questioned the degree to which our understandings of biogenetic relations can be said to have been truly revised, showing that the application of assisted reproductive technologies is itself informed by traditional notions of kinship (Levine, 2008; Thompson, 2005), and that the nuclear family ideal remains a strong notion within the realms of reproduction and parenting (Cutas and Chan, 2012, p. 5). The question of novelty and of how much repro-ductive technologies actually serve to influence or change our understandings of kinship, remains an area of theoretical and empirical debate.

Despite the shared characteristics within the new kinship studies presented earlier, the field remains diverse and continues to draw on different traditions. In a broad categorization of the field, Edwards outlines two main approaches which she terms post-structural (post Leví-Straussian) and post-constructivist (post-Schneiderian). The post-structural approach focuses on the construction of culture as mediated through language; on the 'syntagmatic relations between concepts' and within this approach, it is possible analytically to place 'biological facts' in brackets. The post-constructivist approach, on the other hand, sees 'natural facts' as produced in sociocultural contexts, and kinship as consisting of 'heterogeneous elements' in which 'the context (and intention) determines which of these will be deployed and brought to the fore in a particular instance. The emphasis here is on how kinship is "done"' (2009, p. 17). On reflection, the main difference seems to lie in the various emphases placed on discourse in relation to materiality and in whether or not 'biological facts' are placed in brackets.

I will return to this question when discussing Butler and Haraway, both of whom can be said to thematically represent the two different approaches. Despite the intersections between these two broad categories, this research is mainly positioned within the post-constructivist approach and the focus on 'doing' kinship, in which both the social and biological aspects of kinship are explored in relation to the ways in which family and kinship are practised, and their meaning negotiated by the interviewees in this study. As I will discuss in the next section – and in keeping with the biographical method applied (see Appendix 1) – the doing of family and kinship might underline an element of choice, but they nonetheless are dependent on distinct sociocultural and structural contexts.

2.2.2 *'Doing Family'*

The view of kinship as something that is 'made', in the sense that kinship relations can be transformed and assume new forms of relatedness, has also increasingly preoccupied researchers within the field of family sociology. For instance, the 'family practices approach' developed by David Morgan and the 'family of choice' model represent strands within family sociology that address the ways that people actually *do* family. These traditions do not seek to dismiss or reject the aspect of 'given' but – akin to the new kinship studies – they focus on the interlinkage between both dimensions (May, 2015).

Whereas Chapter 1 in this book merely discusses empirical changes in family life, this section explores two theoretical approaches within the field of family studies, which have sought to comprehend such changes conceptually. The influential family practices approach, developed by David Morgan, sought to shift focus from ideal to real family structures. Then, rather than determining family life against ideal versions of family life, Morgan argued that we should 'focus on how people *do* family' (May, 2015, p. 475). A single focus on 'the family', says Morgan, is likely to use the nuclear family model as point of reference, consequently missing the complexity and multiplicity of family formations, which cannot only be confined within a narrow definition of kin (i.e. established through biology, marriage or lineal descent). Morgan moreover points to the fluid nature of family relations, which are likely to change over time and in different contexts, constantly pushing the boundaries between family and 'non-family' (May, 2015, p. 482; Morgan, 2011).

Other features of the family practice approach include its attentiveness to everyday practices; a focus on social processes and how social relations are enacted as well as how family practices interlink with other sets of practices, for instance in relation to gender and class practices. While the focus on 'doing' and 'social action' might connote unrestrained agency to the detriment of structure, family practices should be viewed not as 'free-floating', but embedded in wider structural contexts. Taking inspiration from the theoretical work of Bourdieu, Morgan also points to the often unconscious enactment of practices and relations and hence to the reproduction of relations as certain structures 'within which these practices have meaning' (Morgan, 2011, p. 2). It is often not until problems emerge or breaches happen (e.g. by divorce) that the status of kin (as opposed to non-kin) are consciously considered. Moreover, family practices are not necessarily positive per se, nor are they a de facto matter of choice (May, 2015). In general, the family practices approach draw on a relational approach where the starting point of analysis in terms of social (family) life is one of social relations rather than the individual or society as pre-existing units (Morgan, 2011).

The family of choice model bears strong similarities to the new kinship studies in addressing the *given* vis-à-vis *made*, in establishing family and kinship. In this regard, the coining of the term 'family of choice' was an attempt to extend the definition of family beyond that of the heterosexual two-parent constellation to include and recognize the many ways in which kin and non-kin relations figure in individuals' family formations. Originally formulated on the basis of studies in same-sex relationships from the 1990s onwards (in particular in Weston's study from 1991), the increasing emergence of LGBT families and families constituted by means of reproductive technologies has only sustained the importance of discussing the formation of family and kinship in terms of the influence of biogenetic and social relations. Changes in family constellations and our understandings of them have also been reflected in legislative changes to, for example, the legality of same-sex marriage. As May further points out, the issue of 'who gets to claim family' remains important and is 'often linked to legal, socio-cultural and economic rights and benefits' (2015, p. 483).

The broader 'doing family' approach can – with its more general focus on the fluid, processual and relational nature of family life – form a theoretical basis to better understand how the interviewed women in this book conceive of and build solo mother families by means of donor conception. Embarking upon solo motherhood entails conscious reflections about how family and kin are to be defined, but we must also regard the decision to become a solo mother as one that is shaped in the complex processes that interlink chosen life plans with available life chances and options (agential and structural possibilities and constraints). Experienced family practices are situated in biographical as well as sociocultural contexts; there is potential tension between the private and the political, within the individual themselves and in the potential duality between ideal expectations and lived realities.

2.3 Identity: Narrative, Gender and Genetics

There is no single overarching story of genetics and identity. Each of the multiple identities that an individual or group may adopt is shaped in the specific environment characterized by a particular configuration of social and technical resources and structured by particular interests, expectations and power relations. Identities have a public and a personal side, and are negotiated in the interplay of individuals, others and institutions that is at once informed by relevant laws, institutions, ideologies and beliefs, yet necessarily responsive to social change and to the influence and agency of individuals and groups.

–Hauskeller et al. (2013, p. 883)

Following the Human Genome Project and its effort to ground explanations of human behaviour in genetics only, social scientists have challenged this effort and questioned the extent to which genetics can serve as an explanatory apparatus for human behaviour and existence. As such, in their scepticism, social scientists have studied 'the myriad ways in which actors draw upon and interpret genetic knowledge as part of their identity-making processes' (Hauskeller et al., 2013, p. 875). How individuals resist or draw on biogenetic knowledge as part of their identity formation is closely related to the discussion of how our genetic thinking influences our kinship thinking and vice versa (see also Nordqvist and Smart, 2014). Identities are shaped in different social processes and in relation to others, and the importance we attach to biogenetic knowledge and inheritance interlinks with our understanding of family and kinship formation.

Genetics may be viewed as a power instrument in the more disciplinarian sense, or 'as enabling new social forms of identity struggles' (Hauskeller et al., 2013, p. 879) in a way that resembles the familiar dualistic discussion of determinism versus voluntarism, or structure versus agency. Such consequences for the enactment of identities have, for instance, been discussed in the work of different social theorists such as Anthony Giddens and Judith Butler. Despite their different approaches to the construction of identities, with Giddens emphasizing the matter of choice over constraint (both in terms of discourse and (body) materiality), both still regard that identities are formed and substantiated within social interaction and both see identities 'as the product of power relations [at where] individual power lies in adopting and living those conditions' (Hauskeller et al., 2013, p. 877). Butler's performative theory on (gender) identity, which will be addressed next, mediates between seeing the individual or subject as both constituted and constitutive and hence in a continual process of becoming, but within a specific discursive, material and historical context.

2.3.1 Individual and Collective Identification

The idiom of identity is well-known and well used both within the academic lingua franca and in our everyday speech. In their famous review of the concept, Brubaker and Cooper argue that the ambiguity, the profusion of meanings attached to the idiom of identity and its 'reifying connotations' (2000, p. 34) has left the idiom without much explanatory force as an analytical concept. In the strong sense of the idiom, identity is taken to express an essentialist and fixed understanding that emphasizes a 'fundamental sameness' across persons and over time (2000, p. 8). By contrast, in the soft sense, the constructivist definition of identity as multiple, fluid and ever changing dilutes the concept according to the authors and renders an understanding of for example, congealed self-understandings and the power of external categorizations difficult. To bypass the tenuous analytical foundation of the concept, Brubaker and Cooper suggest a number of related but specified sets of terms that are not imbued with the same broad and ambiguous connotations as the idiom of identity.

The term of identification, the authors suggest, emphasize the agents that 'do the identifying'. The active form of the verb furthermore underlines the processual and dynamic character of identifying oneself and others, and does not necessarily imply sameness across individuals. The term takes into account the contextual and situational character of self- and other-identification while also allowing for more stable identifications over time. Importantly, identification does not need to only include an 'identifier' such as an individual or institution, but may be more indirectly done by cultural narratives and various discourses that influence individuals' world views and meaning-making. Moreover,

> 'Identification' calls attention to complex (and often ambivalent) *processes*, while the term 'identity', designating a *condition* rather than a *process*, implies too easy a fit between the individual and the social.
>
> –Brubaker and Cooper (2000, p. 17)

Self-understanding is another term suggested as an alternative to that of identity. It refers to 'a situated subjectivity' in the meaning of 'one's sense of who one is, of one's social location, and of how (given the first two) one is prepared to act' (2000, p. 17). Again this term takes into consideration the contextual and changeable nature of how one understands oneself, even though such understandings may come across as stable. Furthermore, the term implies neither sameness nor difference but is able to capture conceptions of self in a more precise way than in the use of the broad concept of identity. Yet, the term of self-understanding does not capture external identifications and classifications of an individual but merely the persons' own understanding of self, even though perceived external identifications are always part of how one understands oneself.

One's self-understanding(s) also include a sense of belonging to certain distinct groups and in this regard the concept of collective identities may imply either a strong 'groupist' or 'loosely affiliative' sense of self-understanding (2000, p. 20). To analytically specify the sense of group-belonging to account for both tight and loose affiliations, Brubaker and Cooper suggest differentiating between the concepts of commonality (sharing of attributes), connectedness (relational ties), which separately or combined may lead to groupness (belonging to a distinct and confined group). The objective with the differentiation of terms is to enable a more nuanced analysis of the many ways in which we enter into and ascribe meaning to different affiliations. In regard to this research, such a differentiation also acts as an analytical reminder not to treat the group of solo mothers in this study (and in general) as a single bounded group or to approach solo motherhood as a pre-defined category (see e.g. May, 2004) in focusing only on commonalities rather than also on internal differences.

A complete dismissal of the concept of identity seem too drastic, given its recognizable and widespread use, and even though it manifests as a broad and fluffy concept, the critique of being caught up in the pitfalls of either essentialism or relativism when applying the concept of identity – as Brubaker and Cooper put forward – seem overemphasized. I agree that one needs to specify one's concepts and be well aware of the explanatory force such concepts provide. Also, in keeping with the constructivist and situated approach of this study, the processual and dynamic focus in the sense of 'doing' rather than 'being', which in particularly is inherent in the concepts of identification and self-understanding, offer a set of analytical concepts through which to explore how the women in this research identify as solo mothers (if this is the case) and how potential changes in their self-understandings and meaning-making manifest biographically in relation to motherhood and fertility treatment, among other experiences and turning points. As for the critical claims of the concept of identity as an analytical heuristic, I argue that several approaches engender a processual and dynamic analytical framework without falling into the above-mentioned pitfalls, despite the fact that they are based on the concept of identity.

The processes of identification are also central to the model proposed by Richard Jenkins (2008). Contrary to Brubaker and Cooper, Jenkins proposes a synthesized model to explain the constitution of individual and collective identities. His 'internal-external dialectic of identification' (Jenkins, 2008, p. 40) unites internal and external processes of definition in accounting for the interaction of the individual and the collective. Each are mutually interdependent; as Jenkins argues, our 'individual and collective identity are as much an interactional product of "external" identification by others as of 'internal' self-identification' (2008, p. 200).

This perception is to be understood according to three different analytical orders; the individual order of embodied individuals highlights that our selves are socially constructed through processes of socialization and are always a matter of both internal and external self-identification as 'we can't see ourselves at all without also seeing ourselves as other people see us' (2008, p. 41). The interaction order refers to human interaction and mediates between the individual and institutional level. Identity is processual and interactional, constituted and validating in the presence of others. Drawing on concepts from Erving Goffman, Jenkins emphasizes 'the performative aspect of identity' (2008, p. 42); in interactions with others, we present ourselves and try to manage the impression we send (impression management) and we try to control how the situation is defined (see Goffman, 1992). The institutional order includes the more established and organized ways of life. At this level, Jenkins analytically locates the processes of collective identification, and he makes a distinction between internal 'group identification' and external 'categorization' (Jenkins, 2008, p. 43). While the first covers how a group defines itself, the latter refers to how others (including institutions) identify and categorize the group. Here too, Jenkins underlines the dialectic relation between the two and the constant manifestations of the drawing of boundaries, power struggles and strategic actions taking place over the allocation of identity positions in the production and reproduction of identities.

The approaches to identification processes proposed by Brubaker/Cooper and Jenkins share many similarities. Yet, whereas Jenkins emphasizes the internal-external dialectic processes of identification in offering a more integrated framework for understanding the complex processes of individual-society inter-play, Brubaker and Cooper offer a set of more specified analytical concepts to explore identification and group affiliations. Combined, they provide a solid basis for exploring identity matters. Nevertheless, to further unfold the performative aspect of identity, this third theoretical mapping will also draw upon the works of Judith Butler.

2.3.2 Butler on Performativity, Gender and Identity

To revert again to Judith Butler's influential theories on gender, sexuality and identity, this section introduces Butler's concept of performativity. A key idea in Butler's work includes the aspect of 'doing gender' in the sense that gender is something one does and not something one is. In this regard, the creation of gender, identity and subject must be understood as 'an ongoing discursive practice [which is] open to intervention and resignification' (Butler, 1999, p. 43). Butler's social constructivist and poststructuralist anchorage manifest in her anti-essentialist theories on gender as social constructions that are shaped within existing and dominating discourses. Hence, gender and other identity catego-rizations are constituted through the materialization of regulating norms and practices and produced through discourse (Butler, 1993). In *Gender Trouble* (1999), Butler critiqued existing gender research for reproducing gender cate-gories within a 'heterosexual matrix' that presupposes a sex-gender division (i.e. the division of sociocultural gender from biological gender). This binary distinction serves to view biological categories of man versus woman as being equal to the masculine man and the feminine woman in naturalizing a hetero-normative ideal of sexuality and identity (Butler, 1999). Butler also made a significant critique of the strands within feminism that viewed the 'woman' as a universal subject and, more broadly, aimed to deconstruct identity categoriza-tions that come to be viewed as naturally-given and fixed and that may cause exclusion and inequality. Butler's transgression of the sex-gender distinction was interpreted by many as an attempt to negate body materiality in perceiving gender, and particularly, as something one could easily perform and change at will. This criticism and the issue of body materiality was addressed in *Bodies that Matter* (1993) in where Butler also refined her theory of performativity.

> Performativity must be understood not as a singular or deliberate 'act', but, rather, as the reiterative and citational practice by which discourse produces the effects that it names.
> –Butler (1993, p. 2)

The performative constitution of cultural norms both enables and limits our actions and the ways in which we continually 'do' gender through the gestures and stylistics of our bodies. In this regard we constantly perform ourselves in the way we strategically present our self to others and in the way we act (Butler, 2004). However, Butler draws a metaphorical parallel to a theatre play in the sense that the performing of a play necessitates both an existing script as well as individual actor interpretations in order for the play to work (Butler, 1988). It is not free play, in the same way as identity categorizations are not just a matter of individual choice.

Butler makes a very central distinction between performativity and performance. Performance is an important aspect of performativity and it refers to the active performance or self-presentation of ones' gender, for instance, that takes place in social processes and interactions (see also Goffman, 1992). Such actions are not to be perceived as single events but as an ongoing citational praxis and a repetition of cultural norms through which gender becomes 'an effect of culturally regulated, discursive practices which, by the very process of regulation, create that which they regulate' (Højgaard, 2012, p. 288). Gender, along with other identity categorizations, is not a pre-given fact according to Butler, but the repetition and cementation of identity norms can make them appear as such.

On the one hand then, we become subjects within discursive and normative expectations which stipulate our possibilities for action. At the same time, we are also constituted as subjects by negotiating and challenging such possible subject positions (Butler, 1999). Butler's focus on 'doing' rather than 'being' adds to the theoretical framework by shifting the main discussion about nature and culture to the individual level, exploring its influence on identity formation while simultaneously challenging 'naturalized' identity categorizations potentially related to motherhood and womanhood, among other topics.

While Butler, like Haraway, attempts to transgress the nature/culture dichotomy (materiality/discourse), Butler primarily maintains a social-constructivist approach to discursive practices that does not specifically regard the 'agency of bodily matter' in contrast to Haraway (Lykke, 2010, p. 120). In this regard, Haraway pays more attention to material processes and perceives the body as a living fact, a continually moving and active matter beyond complete control. Both Butler and Haraway's approach to identity as the product of material and discursive processes add to the ambition of this study to explore the entanglements of reproductive practices with processes of identity construction.

The theoretical and analytical approach to identification processes presented in this third mapping is in keeping with the study's narrative approach to identity (see Appendix 1). Analytically, the aim is not to search for the true and fixed person behind the text, but rather to explore how identities are constructed and presented through the narrative accounts provided. Again, identities are perceived as processual and dynamic, created 'in the stories individuals tell of themselves, situating themselves in relation to other individuals and social structures' (May, 2001, p. 69). Still, in the course of narration, individuals seek to convey a meaningful and coherent story (and identity) in interlinking 'who they are now, how they came to be, and where they think their lives may be going in the future' (McAdams and McLean, 2013, p. 233). Furthermore, in the narrative approach to identity, the individual and the sociocultural is highly interwoven (Horsdal,

2012, p. 100). In several ways then, the concept of identity comes to function as a prism through which to explore the lived experiences of solo motherhood and the implications of assisted reproduction.

2.4 Productive Theoretical Interlinkages

This chapter has combined and presented three main theoretical perspectives or 'mappings' that serve to inform and orient the empirical analysis in this book and that may serve as a basis for more general understandings of the empirical manifestations of 'doing' in terms of identity, gender, family and kinship formation as a continuing negotiation of normalization and naturalization processes.

The first mapping have included feminist theoretical concepts related to the sociocultural implications of reproductive technologies. The individual, social and political implications of medically assisted reproduction have and continue to preoccupy feminist scholars, and the section outlines how the biogenetic and social aspects of reproduction (nature/culture distinction) have been theorized differently depending on whether one for instance adopts a radical feminist or social-constructivist approach. This mapping also discusses contributions from Donna Haraway and Charis Thompson, who seek to transgress the nature/culture distinction by integrating the interdependence of both sociocultural discourse and biological materiality. This dialectic, dynamic and situated approach provides a weighty source of inspiration to explore the experience, meaning and use of assisted reproduction and its influence on reproductive practices and processes of normalization and identity and kinship construction. The second mapping have outlined theoretical concepts within the field of new critical kinship theory and theories on 'doing family'. In the wake of innovations within the field of assisted reproduction and the destabilization of the biological foundation for establishing kinship, the theories included in the second mapping address the complex ways in which kinship emerges as both something 'given' and something 'made' (Carsten, 2004, p. 9). The third mapping continued with the recurring theme of nature versus culture (materiality/discourse) but turned to its implications for identity formation in order to explore how subject positions are adopted, challenged and resisted as they come across in the women's biographical narratives. Moreover, through the presentation of narrative and social identity theory, a processual and dynamic approach to identity formation is adopted in this study, in which the individual and sociocultural are perceived as highly intertwined.

Setting the analytical division between the three mappings aside, the objective has been to explore the interdisciplinary transgressions represented by several of the scholars, and further promote the intersections between them in order to create a productive framework for exploring the empirical implications of medically assisted reproduction. In order to examine questions such as what characterizes the lived experience of relatedness in solo mother families or how the process of fertility treatment influences the life-planning/biographical revisions made by the women in this study, combined understandings from all three mappings appear relevant as they add to the understanding and illustration of the interrelations between relatedness, identity, contexts and technology. In addition to the dynamic and processual nature of the theoretical concepts and approaches included, all dismiss the clear nature/culture binary and seek instead to explore how social and biogenetic aspects interact and substantiate each other in reproducing and disrupting established practices of reproduction and kinship. The following chapters in this book presents the empirical findings of solo motherhood as to how biological and social aspects are variously intertwined when forming different kind of relatedness, exploring the question, among others, of when and why more 'naturalized' kinship and family categories are reproduced and when they are reconfigured within existing sociocultural contexts.

Chapter 3

Getting Access to Fertility Treatment: Governing the 'Natural Order of Life'

The rise of assisted reproductive technologies (ARTs) has increasingly destabilized the boundary between nature and culture and given rise to caused legal and political measures to re-establish a social order by defining 'normal' practice. National and international legislative processes have reflected a fear of the possible risks and misuses which these technologies ensue. At the same time, the technological developments have also continually helped to redefine and stretch the limits of our normative understandings of natural facts and given rise to new understandings of procreation and family formation (Franklin, 1993; Inhorn and Birenbaum-Carmeli, 2008, see Chapter 1).

Danish parliamentary debates on the rights of single and lesbian women to access medically assisted reproduction (MAR) in the public health care system serve as a central example of how this line has been redefined through complex legislative policy processes, leading to the production of new MAR legislation. Through critical frame analysis, this chapter seeks to provide a contextual understanding of the political environment of the governing of MAR in terms of access to these technologies. Hence, it focuses attention on the political and discursive context of legislating assisted reproduction in Denmark. In 2007, single women and lesbian women were granted access to MAR and fertility treatment in public clinics, and this change of legislation has significantly influenced the growing trend of forming solo mother families. This chapter begins by outlining access to MAR and the distinct regulation of gamete donation within a greater European context. It then maps the Danish MAR policy landscape and discusses recent legislative developments in terms of donor conception, among here the introduction of the distinctive Danish two-way donor system in 2012 and the legislative right to double donation introduced in 2018. The chapter then delves into a detailed analysis of the policy transformations that have taken place in Denmark regarding MAR access and finally, the chapter discusses the two main discursive changes found to have taken place. First, 'new family' formations such as solo mother families are increasingly portrayed and represented in positive and inclusive terms, and second, a normalization of reproductive technologies has emerged. The chapter theorizes reproduction as an area of tension between the private and political, and argues that an emerging new governing rationality can

Lived Realities of Solo Motherhood, Donor Conception
and Medically Assisted Reproduction, 55–75
Copyright © 2021 Tine Ravn
Published under exclusive licence by Emerald Publishing Limited
doi:10.1108/978-1-83909-115-520211005

be identified that reflects new biopolitical forms of regulation, risks and subject constructions in accordance with the concept of ethopolitics.

3.1 European Context: Diverse MAR Regulation and Legislation

Within the last decade, MAR regulation in Europe has increased and almost all European countries have now implemented some kind of legislation. Many countries also supplement their MAR governance with voluntary guidelines. A 2008 European Commission directive has established that patients may travel to other countries to obtain treatment – most often designated as 'cross-border reproductive care (CBRC)', even in cases where fertility treatment procedures are against the national regulations of patients' domestic countries. Hence, the main reasons for travelling abroad for treatment have been found to be restrictive regulation, access limitations such as wait times and the quality of treatment. Common EU regulation exist in relation to the application of tissues and cells and for the screening of infections as introduced in the Tissue and Cell Directives from 2004 and 2006. Still, notwithstanding the freedom of movement concerning treatment, no common EU legislation exist on MAR and all EU member states are allowed to adopt their own legislation on assisted reproduction (ESHRE, 2017; Calhaz-Jorge et al., 2020; Shenfield et al., 2010). Differences in cross-country MAR legislation are attributable to variation in cultural, religious, political, financial and social conditions, and primarily concern embryo selection (particularly regarding genetic screening) and preimplantation genetic diagnosis (PGD); egg donation and embryo freezing; surrogacy; donor anonymity and eligibility and access criteria such as age and sexual orientation (ESHRE, 2017; IFFS, 2019). European countries differ as to whether marriage or a stable relationship is required to access MAR. Within the last decade, an increasing number of European countries seem to have loosened their restrictions in this regard, with many countries reporting that no such restrictions are in place. Notable exceptions include Czech Republic, France, Italy, Lithuania, Montenegro, Romania, Serbia, Slovenia, Switzerland and Turkey. Variation also exist among the European countries in whether they allow access to treatment for single women and/or female couples. With regard to access for single women, 31 out of 43 European countries provide treatment whereas 18 out of 43 countries offer treatment to female couples. Countries that grant access to single women include Belgium, Finland, Greece, Bulgaria, the Netherlands, Portugal, Spain and the UK. By contrast, countries which have implemented a more restrictive regulation, excluding single women from accessing treatment, include Italy, France, Switzerland, Turkey, Croatia and Austria (in Austria female couples can be treated). For the remaining Scandinavian countries, Norway have until recently only allowed lesbian women in relationships to access fertility treatment and precluded single women. From July 2020, single women are also offered MAR. Sweden changed its legislation in 2016 on MAR to include single women for treatment if they are below the age of 40 (Calhaz-Jorge et al., 2020; Präg and Mills, 2017; IFFS, 2019; Volgsten and

Schmidt, 2019; HelseNorge, 2020). Factors such as age restrictions and funding and reimbursement policies also mark variation across countries. Präg and Mills (2017) finds that the utility of ARTs interlinks with affordability, costs and age norms for motherhood. For instance, countries such as Denmark, Spain and Slovenia offer treatment covered through national health plans and they are among the countries with the highest level of ART utilization.

As encompassed within the concept of cross-border reproductive care, reproductive technologies cross borders and national contexts. Denmark is a popular and known destination for single and lesbian women pursuing fertility treatments abroad, either due to restricted national regulations in their countries of origin and/or reduced cost and waiting times. Women who travel to Denmark for treatment come from a number of European countries such as France, the UK and Switzerland, with a notable share travelling from Sweden and Norway (Shenfield et al., 2010; Bajekal, 2019). According to numbers provided by the Danish Health Data Authority, in the period from 2011 to 2019, around 2,000 single women living abroad travelled to Denmark each year to undergo fertility treatment.[1] Furthermore, with Cryos International, Denmark hosts the world's largest sperm bank and it exports sperm to all over the world, in particular to other European countries, which import more than 90% of Danish sperm (Andreassen, 2018; Bajekal, 2019).

The availability and advancement of reproductive technologies are of general interest to many, included policymakers due to the technologies' positive effect on completed fertility and the 'potential lever for raising fertility rates in Europe' (Präg and Mills, 2017, p. 291; Sobotka et al., 2008). In this regard, Denmark constitutes an interesting case for investigation and comparison. While developments have taken place in equity and accessibility to assisted reproduction, MAR practices across Europe are still marked by great heterogeneity as to registry databases, fertility treatment outcomes and the obtainability of techniques (Calhaz-Jorge et al., 2020). Consequently, the broader issue of equity in access in terms of domestic and cross-country variance, and the implications for practices and policy-making, remain an important issue that is highly intertwined with that of cross-border reproductive care, 'transparency in the governance of ART' (Baía et al., 2021) and the quality of treatment.

3.2 The Danish Policy Landscape of MAR

In Denmark, MAR is regulated through the 'Act on Assisted Reproduction in connection with Treatment, Diagnosis and Research etc.' (Ministry of Health, no. 902 of 23 August 2019). It stipulates and sets limitations for 'when, to whom and how medically assisted treatment can be offered (couples, single women, age limits, use of unmodified egg- and sperm cells)'. The law also stipulates

---

[1] These numbers were extracted from the Danish IVF-Register and provided by the Danish Health Data Authority upon personal request. The figures concerning Danish single women in fertility treatment are displayed in the introduction to this book.

requirements for treatment information and informed consent (Danish Patient Safety Authority, 2020). The following section details the trajectory of the law in terms of access, tracing the path from the restrictions on access to treatment that were enforced in 1997, to the lifting of the restrictions in 2007, whereas this section outlines the main changes of MAR regulation of particular relevance to solo motherhood vis-à-vis fertility treatment. Specific age limitations and funding/reimbursements policies are included in Chapter 5 on 'Undergoing Fertility Treatment'.

Prior to 2012, only anonymous sperm donation were allowed to be used in medically-run clinics. With the revision on sperm donation in 2012, a new identity-release donor option was introduced and following this change in legislation, single women and couples embarking upon fertility treatment with donor sperm could now choose between either an anonymous, non-anonymous or known donor (for specific details on the Danish sperm donor model, see Chapter 7).

Denmark allows for egg donation which, like sperm donation, can be either anonymous or non-anonymous. In 2006, due to shortage of donated eggs, the limitation on egg-donors being women undergoing in vitro fertilization (IVF) treatment themselves was lifted, thus allowing all women to become donors. Still, potential egg donors have to meet certain age (<35) and health requirements. The change in legislation helped to remedy the shortage but not enough to meet the demands. Hence, monetary compensation for egg donors has been raised in several sittings, recently in 2016 to 7,000 Dkk (940 EUR) per donation. In 2018, Denmark allowed for double donation, where medical circumstances deemed it useful or necessary, either due to infertility issues or to the potential risk of passing on inherited diseases to potential offspring. Double donation can only be offered if at least one of the donors is non-anonymous (Herrmann, 2018; Ministry of Health, 2020a). Within the public health care system, women can freeze and store their eggs and embryos if it relates to fertility or medical treatment. Cryo-preservation of eggs is only possible for women who intend to postpone potential motherhood until later in life – a praxis termed 'social egg freezing' (Baldwin, 2019) – at private fertility clinics. Recently, the five-year storage limit has been debated on the basis of a citizen proposal suggesting to extend the period of storage. As no health professional reasons serves as a rationale for a specific five-year storage period, the Danish parliament has agreed to prolong the period of egg freezing until the woman in question reaches the age of 46 which is the age limit for assessing fertility treatment in private clinics. The change will come into effect in 2021 (Ministry of Health, Guideline no. 9351 of 26 May 2015; Ministry of Health, 2020b).

3.3 The Policy Trajectory from Restrictive to Permissive on Access to MAR

In the Danish political debates on equal access to assisted reproduction single and lesbian women are referred to in a more or less interchangeable manner and – in contrast to other country models – the two do not differ in terms of legal requirements and conditions. The chapter addresses both groups, but nevertheless focuses on the representation of single women in the debates (keeping in mind that the categories are not mutually exclusive).

The birth of the first Danish child conceived by means of IVF in 1983 triggered a heated political debate as the new reproductive possibilities had more or less surreptitiously emerged without any formal legislative regulation or public debate in the Danish context. Until the first bill (L200 on 'artificial insemination regarding medical treatment, diagnostics and research etc.') was introduced in 1996 by the Minister of Health (Social Democratic Government), with the intention to regulate and visualize practice within the area, the field of biotechnology was directed by 'law on bio-medical research projects' and different guidelines. However, increased awareness of, and a concomitant moral panic about the possibly negative consequences of this new technology, created a need for political regulation. Previous regulation did not include any formal differentiation in access to assisted reproduction, however, in practice this did not apply as the counties in charge of hospitals only offered infertility treatment to heterosexual couples in stable relationships. Single and lesbian women were therefore referred to private clinics for treatment. The first bill (L200) entailed no instructions for changing this practice, nor did the following bill (L5), which was a resubmission of the first one introduced the same year. Nevertheless, an amendment suggesting that only married women or women in a marriage-like relationship be allowed access to medical reproductive treatment was introduced in the 2nd reading of the debate – by a group of MPs from the Social Democratic Party – and a majority from both government and opposition voted for this motion in 1997 and the subsequent § 3 in what became law no. 460. The paragraph entailed a direct ban on any doctors – in the public as well as in the private health care system – offering assisted reproduction to single and lesbian women. The debate continued and several attempts to alter this paragraph were set in motion the following year by MPs across the political spectrum but were not realized. Several years later, in 2002, MPs from the Red-Green Alliance tried again unsuccessfully to abrogate the paragraph (L118) and in 2005, continued the efforts with a resubmission of the same amendment, with a similar result (L115).

As mentioned in the introduction, in January 2007 lesbian and single women obtained the same right to fertility treatment in the public health care system as heterosexual women, who were married or living in a married-like relationship (law 535 of 8 June 2006). Hence, doctors in both the public and private health care system were allowed to contribute to assisted reproduction for all women, regardless of marital status or sexual orientation. Again, the actual sequence of events leading up to the passing of this law and the preceding bill (L151) displayed a rather peculiar trajectory. The original bill did not include any alterations of the paragraph, but served to prolong the duration of storage of frozen embryos from two to five years, loosen restrictions on oocyte donation as well as establish criteria for an assessment of parent suitability in connection with infertility treatment. Yet, the bill introduced by the Minister of the Interior and Health (liberal-conservative government) included a memorandum on the issue of women's equal access to assisted reproduction to function as a basis for further debate in the readings, as this issue had been the pivot point of previous debates. An actual amendment seeking to revoke the paragraph was put forward during the second reading by a unified opposition and barely passed by means of a small minority (six MPs) from the Liberals. The final bill (L151) was passed with 86 votes in favour and 61 votes against. However, the majority of politicians from the political party which originally formulated and introduced the bill (the Liberals), then voted against it as a result of the passing of the amendment giving single and lesbian women equal access to assisted reproduction.

In 1996, a majority of political parties released their MPs from the party line due to the ethical character of the subject matter, and this was mirrored in the split both within and across parties. In contrast to this, the voting in 2006 was characterized by a greater level of unity as the oppositional parties had implemented party discipline in this area, leaving only the Liberals with internal disagreements in relation to policy making within the area of assisted reproduction. The greater unity among the opposing parties probably had some effect on the vote, as did the appointment of new political spokespersons, but arguably, these were effects only in so far they influenced and were influenced by emerging discursive changes (Parliament records; Parliamentary News; Bryld, 2001; Bryld and Lykke, 2000; Lykke and Bryld, 2006; Petersen, 2007; Hoffmann-Hansen, 2006).

The policy trajectory concerning access from restrictive to permissive by law (Engeli, 2009, p. 57) has not been a straightforward process as described above. If a policy issue is framed as a moral issue and at the same time characterized by plural values or a 'clash of moral absolutes', the policy response will often lead to failure in decision-making (Engeli and Varone, 2011, pp. 246–248). The Danish case could be interpreted along these lines; the strong political incentives of revoking restricted access did not impact the political agenda much, as the incumbent government did not wish to make decisions within this value-laden area. Furthermore, the procedure of only including a memorandum in the introduction of the bill substantiates this reluctance to deal with a policy subject that caused disagreement across and within political parties.

Despite the level of political debate on this policy issue, the involvement of non-party actors has been modest. In general, institutions like the Council of Ethics and the Centre of Human Rights had an impact on the process without politicizing the issue. In terms of access to MAR, LGBT Denmark was active during this period of debate and legislation, too (Albæk et al., 2012). It has not, however, been a prevalent issue for feminist interest parties and individuals, neither within nor outside of parliament. This is presumably due to the turbulent trajectory of the amendment and the fact that the issue of access was never directly submitted for consultation since it was not included in any originally formulated bills. Two other factors also appear pertinent. Firstly, in terms of 'state feminism', Denmark's version is primarily defined according to a 'bottom-up oriented model' rather than an 'institutionalized model' as in Sweden, and unlike the latter, feminist issues have 'never gained ground in the political parties' (Borchorst and Siim, 2008, pp. 210–211). Secondly, as described in the introductory chapter, reproductive technology has been a matter of ambivalence for many feminists since they may help overcome involuntary childlessness, but concurrently add to the reproduction and essentializing of gender expectations to reproduction (Thompson, 2005, p. 55). Hence, the lack of a well-defined policy-cycle and of a coherent and strategic feminist framing within and without parliament can add to the explanation of the limited feminist representation in the agenda-setting process.

3.4 Framing the Two Main Debates through Critical Frame Analysis

The frame analysis presented in this chapter, explores how policy positions are framed and legitimized in the 2006/2007 parliamentary debates on equity of access to MAR using governmentality as a frame of reference. Furthermore, the analysis compares these debates to the debates 10 years earlier (1996/1997) where access to MAR was restricted to married women or women living in a 'marriage-like relationship'. As outlined in the previous section, the process leading up to and following the passing of the law reflected an 'agonistic area' in which conflicts over what counts as truth were played out (Rose, 2003, p. 185). In other words, it revealed conflicting frames at play in the conceptualization of this particular policy issue.

The policy debate on access to MAR took place primarily during two distinct legislative processes; the first in 1996–1997 with the adoption of bill L5 (three prescribed readings), which restricted access to assisted reproduction for single and lesbian women in both the private and public health care systems. The second main debate took place 10 years later in 2006/2007 during the parliamentary debates (3 prescribed readings) which consequently led to bill L152 and a lifting of the former access restrictions. Due to the particular relevance of these key debates, the framing and legitimization of different political positions on access to MAR will be explored through these two main cases. Accordingly, the analysis will focus on the different issue frames (i.e. 'the meaning of a specific policy area' in particular policy debates (Sauer, 2010, p. 194) which were constructed during the debates. Specifically, debate transcripts from each of the six readings serve as data used for analysis.[2] In this regard, the general lack of non-party actors renders an analysis of particular micro-frames (i.e. the positioning of different 'organized ideas' by specific political and non-political actors) (Sauer, 2010, pp. 193–194) less pertinent.

---

[2] A summary of case histories and committee handlings regarding various bills from 1985–1986 to 2003–2004 are to be found electronically in the records of the Parliament at ⟨http://webarkiv.ft.dk/doc.aspx?/samling/arkiv.htm⟩: whereas parliamentary proceedings from this period are only located in printed versions of the records named 'Parliament News' (Folketingstidende). The printed versions were replaced in 2004–2005 with an electronic version, which allows for a download of completed case histories (www.ft.dk). Additionally, information on passed bills is available at retsinformation.dk (court information).

Critical frame analysis provides a useful approach for exploring how political positions are represented and contended in the political debates, how social meanings are shaped within various frameworks and how female and parental identities are negotiated. The critical frame analysis applied in this chapter is informed by the methodological work of Donald Schön and Martin Rein in analysing intractable policy controversies. According to this perspective, frames are viewed as 'policy positions resting on underlying structures of belief, perception, and appreciation' (1994, p. 23), and furthermore, in their definition, 'framing is a way of selecting, organizing, interpreting, and making sense of a complex reality to provide guideposts for knowing, analysing, persuading and acting' (Rein and Schön, 1993, p. 146). Additionally, the analysis is informed by the notion of 'reflexive framing' (Bacchi, 2009). In order to grasp how the cultural framework of which we are part shapes our notions of key concepts, such as parenthood, reflexive framing urges us to tend reflectively to the underlying assumptions and premises that form policy frames and consequently are con- stituents of the foundation for interpretation. Hence, frame analysis provides a valuable tool for the study of the explicit and conscious shaping of arguments ('strategic framing') as well as the more implicit and unconscious understandings which underpin conflicting policy positions and statements (Bacchi, 2009; Wagenaar, 2011). In order to include both explicit and implicit framing, the analysis pays attention to the negotiation and legitimation of frames while also tending to the ideological and normative understandings underlying the policy positions presented in the debates.

Despite the intractable character of policy controversies, frame shifts in 'problem-setting' frames can take place, most likely in response to changed situations over time and as a result of changes in different contexts (denoted nested contexts), within which framing of policy issues always occur. These changes can entail a reframing of the policy issue in question with or without 'frame reflection'. In simpler terms 'frame reflection' and the possible related reframing process happen 'in the course of the participant's conversation with their situation' (Rein and Schön, 1993, p. 163). In this regard, it has furthermore been suggested that at least two disparate processes can ensue from the dynamics of reframing; one, the wish to 'fix belief' can eventually entail a dominant frame to change, as it is challenged by oppositional politics and the changing practices of citizens' daily experiences. Secondly, conventional policy can be challenged; nonetheless it adapts to and copes with these challenges, which does not initially cause reframing; however small adaptations can have unintended consequences, eventually leading to problem redefinition and reframing (Laws and Rein, 2003, pp. 175–176).

The frame analysis in this chapter is based on two analytical strategies. First, directed by a preliminary inductive research strategy, the research process has been empirically driven and founded, based on the principles and procedures of grounded theory methods. Guidelines for engaging in systematic and focused analysis while at the same time applying 'an open, generative, emergent meth- odology', without normatively forcing one's data to fit preconceived theories (Glaser, 1998, pp. 94 and 83) has been a main directive for the qualitative coding procedure. First, the procedures of 'initial' and 'focused' coding as outlined by Charmaz (2006) were applied to the 2006–2007 debate transcripts. The final list of codes was compared to data again and applied to the 1996–1997 debate transcripts to facilitate a systematic and in-depth within-case and cross-case analysis of the two cases.

3.5 Biopolitical Perspectives

Whether or not we should embrace the technological possibilities of assisted reproduction as a society has been a salient element in the two Danish debates on equal access to MAR, especially in terms of where the line between the 'natural' and 'artificial' should be drawn. As one politician states in the 2006 debate:

> Nature sets boundaries. Should Danish legislation also decide the boundaries of nature? We believe not.
> –Birthe Skaarup (the Danish People's Party, DPP, 1st reading, 2006, p. 7)

As pointed out by Lemke (2009, p. 35), a biopolitical frame of reference enables a 'making visible' of boundaries between life and politics as well as between culture and nature. The biopolitical perspective and concept of governmentality have been actualized by Nikolas Rose, who has argued that a biological view of human nature has been influential in recent years; indeed, policy surrounding the matter has largely been concerned with biological issues on the molecular level, reflecting a 'politics of life itself' (Rose, 2001; 2007). This 'politics of life itself' is linked to the biosciences and biological aspects of life as regards reproductive technology, gene therapy and the use of stem cells for medical intervention etc. and is no longer based on natural life or functions as the norm 'against which a politics of life may be judged' (Rose, 2001, p. 17; The Danish Council of Ethics, 2010). Contemporary biopolitics attend to the control and reshaping of the 'vital processes of human existence' (Rose, 2001, p. 1), which, broadly speaking, has led to new forms of regulation, risks and subjectivities (Rose, 2001). Today, biopolitics can be juxtaposed with 'ethopolitics'. According to the latter, individual and political actions and conduct are now governed by morality and ethics, and engaged with 'the quality of life', 'the right to life' and 'the right to choose':

> By ethopolitics, I mean to characterize ways in which the ethos of human existence – the sentiments, moral nature or guiding beliefs of persons, groups, or institutions – have come to provide the 'medium' within which the self-government of the autonomous individual can be connected up with the imperatives of good government.
> –Rose (2001, p. 18)

This autonomy and the range of multiple choices each individual is required to make, in terms of marriage and procreation for instance, entails increased responsibility for one's own self-governing. Alongside this 'liberation', however, political powers seek to form and shape the conduct of individuals in accordance with dominating norms and discourses through various techniques. Authority is internalized, while individuals simultaneously become autonomous and self-determinate subjects. Thus, individuals are obligated to act as autonomous individuals, pursuing self-improvement and optimization through a range of self-realization techniques in order to reach certain objectives (Rose, 2001; 2003; 2007). As demonstrated, this type of politics is not power-neutral or free of moral judgments, as it specifically regulates individuals' way of life according to morality and ethics; however, the space for individual action, self-realization and choice seems broadened while paving the way for new sets of ethical norms regarding the constitution of 'normal'.

3.6 Different Issue Frames at Play in the Debates on Access to MAR

The discussion on how to define and understand natural facts in terms of pro-creation and family formation is a generally recurring issue transcending the related themes discussed in the parliamentary debates. Perceptions of what is considered natural vs. artificial serve as moral and ethical guiding principles for setting legislative boundaries. Decision-making regarding biopolitical questions is, however, not only a matter of technology assessment or compromises between sets of values but also a matter of 'how normative ideas on individual freedom and responsibility function with biological factors' (Lemke, 2009, pp. 39–40). In the debates, these more general, normative ideas function as components underpinning the different political positions represented with various emphases on freedom and responsibility. However, these ideas are entangled in complex ways in attitudes towards procreative choices and different types of reflections on what is perceived as the proper foundation for parenthood – again, depending on various views on life and human nature.

3.6.1 The Debate in 2006: Three Lines of Conflicting Argumentation

In the 2006 debate, the left wing is in favour of the motion to grant access whereas the right wing is against, with the exception of the Liberal Party (L), which is divided between a complete endorsement of the motion (a minority) and a partial endorsement contingent on self-payment.

3.6.1.1 The Best Interest of the Child

This ethical approach also indicates that for a majority of us in the Conservative parliamentary group, it is not particularly decisive

whether the procedure takes place in the public or private auspices; or, moreover, where the bill is sent to. For us, it is now primarily a question of what should be permitted, which norms we want our society to set, which rules should be applied for the utilization of technological possibilities and, finally, what we as a legislative power wish to signal is the ideal – is the best for children.
–Pia Christmas-Møller (The Conservative People's Party, CPP, 1st reading, 2006, p. 12)

A consistent notion throughout the lines of argumentation is that the opponents of the motion seek to argue in favour of the biological nuclear family on the basis of a belief that the best interest of the child is to be raised by both a mother and father and that legislators should not deny future children that possibility. Children should also know their genetic roots. Further argument is made to the effect that nature sets the boundaries for how a child can be conceived (despite technological possibilities) and that single and lesbian women are therefore not entitled or have a right to have a child.

However, we think that when it is discussed, we repeatedly miss the angle that state legislation must not prevent children from having a father. Besides, it is a point from nature's part that it takes a man and a woman to create a child (...) The brave new world moves the borders and consequences for our children, and this is why we say 'no' to the amendments.
–Birthe Skaarup (the Danish People's Party, DPP, 2nd reading, Parliamentary News, 2006, pp. 7611–7612)

Several issues are at stake here. It becomes evident, however, that representatives of the position expressed above wish to sustain a 'natural order' whereby the nuclear family is seen as the ideal family ideology towards which we should be striving. Fears of loss of traditional family values, along with a potential breakdown of the existing social order, are immanent concerns according to this line of argument. As Sarah Franklin has pointed out:

Where the "natural" basis for certain forms of essentialist moralism has been eroded it can easily be reconstructed through other channels, such as the law. The threat to essentialism is thus recuperated in order to re-establish it.
(Franklin, 1993, p. 32)

In other words, the brave new world of procreative options threatens to erode this aforementioned 'natural order', causing MPs from the political right wing to undertake political endeavours to re-establish it through regulatory actions.

What is perceived as the 'normal' grounds of parenting and family formation constitutes the foundation by which the field of actions of single and lesbian women is sought to be governed; in this case, by excluding single and lesbian women from access to reproductive technologies, the argument being that the wellbeing of the potential child takes precedence over the freedom of women's procreative choice – in so far as this does not encompass all women, but single and lesbian women only. The rights of the embryo and best interest of the potential child generally marked the debate among the opponents and pro-ponents of the motion alike. Beneath this issue, however, the question of parental suitability also permeated the debate:

> The unborn child is definitely the weak party, since it is silent and defenseless but still the party which must live with the decisions made by adults; whether the decisions are made by adults in the role of parents or legislators.
> –Pia Christmas-Møller (The Conservative People's Party, CPP, 1st reading, 2006, p. 11)

The 'best interest of the child' is repeatedly highlighted and used as a catchphrase to symbolize an infrangible relation between the child's best interests and the nuclear family. Furthermore, the concept of 'family' is similarly employed in a manner that takes for granted that a family consists of both a (biological) father and mother, thereby discarding family constellations which do not fit this model.

As also expressed in the above-mentioned quotation, the unborn child is represented as the powerless party, which will fall victim to the mistreatment of single and lesbian women if they should be allowed access to reproductive technologies. Furthermore, it is explicitly assumed that having access to both a biological mother and father as role models is the best option for the child to develop their personal identity; and it is thus presupposed that the lack of a potential biological father figure will entail a less happy upbringing and provide less beneficial conditions for the development of a healthy identity. Scientific research stating that there is nothing to substantiate such conclusions – and that children brought up by single and lesbian women thrive just as much as children raised in the 'nuclear' family constellation – is also questioned and disregarded by opponents of the motion;

> Can I just say in relation to those studies that not much research has been performed within this area, and it is highly questionable whether it can be studied at all. Alone the question as to how to construct objective criteria is an object for scientific discussions – an issue which has also caught the attention of the Danish Council of Ethics.
> –Pia Christmas-Møller (The Conservative People's Party, CPP, 1st reading, 2006, p. 13)

Conversely, the proponents continuously refer to the aforementioned research in order to make clear that the life conditions of children are not impaired if they are raised by single or homosexual parents. As the debates and divided recommendations from The Danish Council of Ethics demonstrate (2004, p. 17), this ethical issue precludes one-sided sentiments on the consequences of granting equal access to MAR. Moreover, facts are used inconsistently in the arguments presented, underlining the point that 'data that do not fit within the frame, simply don't make sense to the adherents of the frame' (Wagenaar, 2011, p. 85). The use of scientific research and facts in the debates also substantiate the point made by Schön and Rein (1994, p. 4) that facts, and sometimes the same set of facts, are chosen and interpreted in various ways according to the understandings inherent in the conflicting frames, making policy controversies resistant to resolution.

> Homosexual couples can be just as caring, loving and responsible towards children as others. That children in fact are brought up in such family settings and that they actually – as other children – normally have a safe and loving upbringing are real life facts. However, it is simply not a fact which makes us believe that we should then underpin, institutionalize and set norms for such a pattern whereby the father- or mother figure are deselected beforehand.
> –Pia Christmas-Møller (The Conservative People's Party, CPP, 1st reading, 2006, p. 12)

In a similar vein, the proponents of granting single and lesbian women access to MAR put forward the following argument:

> We have heard that the children of single and lesbian women now thrive in a manner comparable to other children with the same opportunities and same risks. That is why we are very comfortable about the situation if we can achieve completely equal rights.
> –Karen J. Klint (the Social Democrats, SDP, 1st reading, 2006, p. 7)

In this statement, the same fact is presented as in the above-mentioned quotation but framed differently. As opposed to the aforementioned arguments, this opposite view holds that single and lesbian women are as good parents as any and that children raised by single and lesbian women experience just as happy and loving upbringings as children raised in nuclear families. As mentioned, the proponents of the motion substantiate this argument by referring to scientific research within the area and to tangible family demographics in the Danish society in general; children are already and increasingly reared in blended families, parents divorce with the result that children sometimes do not see their fathers and, in other cases yet, some children do not know their biological fathers. Even though it is stated that these latter examples do not necessarily provide the child with optimal conditions, the argument holds that such circumstances and developments cannot be prevented by legislation. Families are constructed in various ways, and parenthood can be understood in distinct manners, as for instance in terms of biological, social, legal and moral parenthood; all of which can imply various parental rights and responsibilities. Thus, a genetic parent who provides gametes consisting of sperm or egg is not necessarily a 'social' parent who raises and cares for the child and is seen socially as being responsible for the child (Brake and Millum, 2012, pp. 2–3).

Where opponents of letting single and lesbian women access MAR define the grounds of parenthood in a monistic manner by attaching importance to biological categorizations, the proponents instead perceive parenthood on the basis of pluralistic relations between individuals, which are not necessarily biological yet still fulfil the responsibilities, functions and purposes of a family. The latter thus accentuates moral agency (e.g. by including the intentions for wanting a child) rather than focusing more explicitly on biology (Peterson, 2005, p. 282; Brake and Millum, 2012, pp. 17–20). Thus, proponents of the motion view the concept of family as a broader concept, including various types of family constellations, thereby also expanding on what is perceived as natural and what constitutes the basis of moral parenthood in terms of rights and responsibilities. One argument in this regard expresses that if the course of nature should be followed, assisted reproduction on the whole should be disregarded, as it already transgresses the boundaries of nature, meaning that nature as such has 'decided' that infertile individuals cannot have children (Kamal Qureshi, Socialist People's Party, SPP, 2nd reading, Parliamentary news, 2006, p. 7612). By questioning the 'nature of the natural' (Lie, 2002, p. 382) in terms of reproduction, the view expresses that granting single and lesbian women access to assisted reproduction is no more natural or unnatural than heterosexual couples' usage of ARTs.

3.6.1.2 Equality and Reproductive Rights

Proponents of the motion also legitimize their position through arguments emphasizing discriminatory elements in the existing legislation and question the basis upon which opponents regard the best interest of the child:

> I do not believe that any of us want to disregard the best interest of the child or the consideration for the child. We just disagree whether considerations for the best interest of the child call for the presence of two sexes.
> –Karen J. Klint (the Social Democrats, SDP, 1st reading 2006, p. 7)

Again, the biological, two-parent family constellation is rendered nonessential, while whether the father figure constitutes an imperative foundation for the wellbeing of a child is also questioned (Bryld and Lykke, 2000). Furthermore, the lack of equal access to assisted reproduction is seen as a discriminatory prohibition, as it excludes specific groups from accessing medical assistance on the basis of their marital status. As also stressed in this regard, heterosexual couples can exercise their right to assisted reproduction in the public health care system without any specific diagnosis, as they are considered involuntarily childless; the argument thus holds that single and lesbian women should be able to access the same assistance – also without any specific diagnosis.

> For me, this is also about a certain form of equality: Equality for women. Regardless of marital status, regardless of what type of relationship you live in, this parliament should implement equality for all women with regards to having children.
> –Lene Hansen (the Social Democrats, SDP, 2nd reading, Parliamentary News, 2006, p. 7612)

This second line of reasoning implies a weighting of women's procreative rights to reproduce, to sexual autonomy and for women to decide over their own bodies. Hence, due to the above-mentioned arguments, it is contended that single and lesbian women should have access to assisted reproduction on the same terms as women living in a heterosexual relationship.

The framework presented above encompasses an ideological conviction and a set of values which accentuates alternative family forms and represents a redefinition of the nature–culture boundary while affecting the normative conceptualization of procreation and parenting. Boundaries for what is perceived as the natural, and thus ideal foundation for parenthood are thus transgressed, as is the presumed essential relationship between biological parenthood (both sexes included) and the wellbeing of children.

Furthermore, the subject position of single and lesbian women in terms of parenthood is constructed differently within this framework, employing a less one-sided articulation of what constitutes a 'normal' mother and woman. For instance, single and lesbian women are also represented as: '...qualified parents, who will bring up some really good and well-functioning children' (Karen J. Klint, the Social Democrats, SDP, 1st reading 2006, p. 7). This highlights the argument that the strong desire to have children, possibly at great expense, could point to 'top-motivated parents, who make a great effort' in terms of parenting (The Danish Council of Ethics, 2004, p. 16). The rationale behind this governing strategy thus appears to operate on a different logic, which does not have the safeguarding of traditional family structures as its core objective. Instead, the rationale appears to be that single and lesbian women should be governed in accordance with new standards for family formation, reflecting an emerging metacultural frame, which normatively guides this policy position. The policy solution of giving women equal access to assisted reproduction does not favour 'liberating' these groups of women to the detriment of the welfare of children, since the underlying rationale entails an equalization and normalization of the above-mentioned family formations with a view to the best interests of children.

3.6.1.3 Health Care Rights and Self-payment

A third but minor central line of argument is also present in the debates, representing the understanding that single and lesbian women are entitled to medical treatment but since they are not to be viewed as ill, they should pay for treatment themselves outside of the public health care system. Here, single and lesbian women are seen as 'juridical subjects whose conduct is to be limited by law' (Roseet al., 2006, p. 85) and who must be governed in consistency with resource prioritizations vis-à-vis individual health care rights. However, the main frame conflict between ideological understandings of parenthood and procreation can be seen as a conflict between a nature frame and a culture frame, which also reflects a political conflict between the left and right wings. Whereas these conflicting normative frames are also represented in the 1996 debate 10 years earlier, the political left-right split is not. Instead, the 1996 policy controversy manifests itself both within and across the entire political spectrum.

3.6.2 Developments over a Decade: Towards New Normative Images of Reproductive Technologies and Procreation

When comparing the debate in 2006 as outlined above with the one in 1996, one substantial feature permeates the latter: the fear of the potential risks and misuses which could follow in the wake of ARTs.

> And then some of us believe that the current development really is a development out over the edge and quite awful; therefore, we would like to dig in our heels and try to steer clear of what some would call 'full steam ahead'.
> –Margrete Auken (Socialist People's Party, SPP, 2nd reading, Parliamentary News, 1997, p. 6368)

> I fear that we are changing our view of human nature towards perceiving one another as things and where we do not perceive one another as human beings.
> –Niels Jørgen Langkilde (The Conservative People's Party, CPP, 2nd reading, Parliamentary News, 1997, p. 6379)

A number of MPs on both sides of the Danish parliament express a fear of a possible depersonalization, technification and objectification of humans if they are to be created in the 'laboratory' to a greater extent. It is not so much the technologies as such but how they can be applied (Balling and Lippert-Rasmussen, 2006, p. 11), which raises the need for extensive governance and a strict technological assessment of the – at the time – new technologies. In addition to responses regarding the establishment of rules within an area which was by and large, left unregulated, much of the 1996 debates are marked by a moral panic as a response to the technological advancements. Lines of argumentation and symbolic markers are based on emotional and normative understandings, insisting that the technological practices must resemble natural processes to the extent possible 'in helping nature along', if the technologies could not be prohibited altogether, as some proposed (cf. Bryld, 2001; Lykke and Bryld, 2006). As expressed in the quotation below, personal sentiments directed the political positions represented:

> It is difficult to give a rational answer as to why the time period for
> [egg] freezing should be one year. It is the thought of the artificial
> which scares me; that you, two or three years after a fertilised egg
> has been frozen, take it out and insert it into the uterus.
> –Henriette Kjær (The Conservative People's Party, CPP,
> 1st reading, Parliamentary News, 1996, p. 247)

A technocentric version of biopolitics is clearly expressed in the quotation as well as in the general debate discussing where to set boundaries between 'what we believe to be right and what we believe to be wrong' (Vibeke Peschardt, the Danish Social-Liberal Party, 1st reading, Parliamentary News, 1996, p. 249).[3] In the early 1996 debate, efforts to maintain clear boundaries between natural and artificial processes through the controlling of technological advances are much more pronounced than in the later debate. In the 2006 debate, the fear and risks ensuing from ARTs have been reshaped and the moral panics have ceased. The technology as such serves much more as an implicit premise for debating access to assisted reproduction, and the regulation of ARTs is primarily discussed in correlation with for whom this technology is designed:

> Nature has decided that two women cannot have children together
> and this is what we rely on, not on the appearance of the new
> technology.
> –Birthe Skaarup (the Danish People's Party DPP, 2nd reading,
> Parliamentary News, 2006, p. 7612)

Such attempts to re-establish the 'natural order of life' (e.g. with regard to 'appropriate' parenthood) draw on different technological presumptions. The establishment in 1996 of restricted access to MAR should be viewed in light of the moral panic fuelling the debate (cf. Bryld, 2001). The attendant insecurity and fear of the unknown increased the effort to limit changes endangering any familiar practices; as one Liberal MP pointed out, granting access to lesbian women would be the beginning of 'a slippery slope', which would entail single women applying ARTs and, somewhere down the road, two homosexual men being able to adopt a child. To legitimize this position of where to say 'stop', the familiar argument of 'naturalness' was used as a generative metaphor and a line of demarcation:

---

[3]A technocentric version of biopolitics is in general concerned with questions regarding whether or not societies should embrace technological possibilities, and how technological practices modify and impact on nature (Lemke, 2009, pp. 35ff).

> Since two lesbian women have no natural chances of having
> children, we say 'no' to offering lesbian women this option.
> –Jørgen Winther (the Liberals, L, 3rd reading, Parliamentary
> News, 1997, p. 7809)

A similar argument is posed by a Social Democrat MP:

> In human behaviour, it is not always possible to succeed in
> ensuring a child a father and a mother, but I believe that when
> making rules for an activity, we should come as close to the natural
> as possible.
> –Hans Peter Baadsgaard (2nd reading, Parliamentary News, 1997,
> p. 6376)

The emphasis on bio-genetic processes in preserving 'normal' family structures resembles understandings inherent in the aforementioned nature frame. In
fact, the same line of argumentation, with regard to the best interest of the child
and consequently the right to both a (biological) mother and father, are also
posed in this early debate. In fact, although composed slightly differently, the
nature frame by far represents the dominant issue frame, as a majority of MPs
across political parties adopt the rationalities and meaning constructions within
this frame.

Compared to the 2006 debate, only a few MPs express the view that single
and lesbian women make just as good parents as heterosexual couples and that
legislation within this area should reflect the diversity of family formations in
society at large. Additionally, a smaller group of MPs suggest allowing single
and lesbian women medical access to insemination (not IVF) in order not to
criminalize medical treatment and avoid a practice of insemination possibly
taking place under 'less safe conditions'. For this group of MPs, the predominant matter is equal healthcare rights rather than equal reproductive rights
between women.

Contrary to the later debate, this oppositional frame never fully unfolds, and
it never comes to represent an actual alternative to the dominant view of
adhering to 'traditional' family formations; partly because the oppositional
frame appears divided in how the policy problem is represented and consequently, in the normative understanding inherent in this frame. Contrary to this,
in 2006, the culture frame manifests itself as a competing policy frame to the
previously predominant nature frame. This could indicate that the proliferation
of MAR and 'new family' formations have given rise to the broader acceptance
and recognition of single and same-sex parenthood as reflected in the political
debate. In other words, changes in the Danish cultural context or the 'metacultural frames' have affected legislation towards new normative images of
reproductive technologies and procreation. Meanwhile, the internal context
for policy framing also changed; some MPs have been replaced and others have
changed their positions on access to assisted reproduction though frame
reflection:

I think times have changed a lot, and I also believe that the concept of family has changed. The concept of family is not what it used to be. (...) I have changed my position on this area. It was me who suggested ten years ago only providing assisted reproduction to married women or women living in a 'marriage-like relationship'. That was what I meant at the time and what I have meant for some years. And back when I said it, the entire Liberal parliamentary group actually meant it.
    –Jørgen Winther (the Liberals, L, 2nd reading, Parliamentary
News, 2006, p. 7608)

Changes over time regarding cultural transformations and shifts in political positions have acted as a catalyst for the reframing of this policy issue. Still, when analysing the later debate, it becomes evident that it can be characterized as an intractable policy controversy impervious to resolution by examination of facts. Furthermore, the formerly dominant nature frame also continued to mark the later debate. Hence, if we are to understand reframing as a complete dismissal of a former dominant frame, then reframing has not occurred in this case.

Still, the introduction of new MAR legislation also emphasized that opposi-tional politics and emerging cultural practices eventually challenged the bio-logized understandings inherent in the nature frame. Interestingly, as the analysis establishes, this did not imply that the culture frame then entered a new dominant position. Developments taking place did influence the altering of the status quo and the discursive construction of 'natural practices' in terms of family forma-tions. However, these transformations are perhaps best viewed according to the notion of 'liminal spaces' as a 'between space' where 'new meaning, new ways of sense making begin to materialize but are not yet realized' (Cobb in Laws and Rein, 2003, p. 205). Whereas the actual legislative practice of giving equal access to MAR was realized, the acceptance of pluralistic family formations was not. Thus, the emerging dynamics of reframing are best described as social change moving towards new normative images of reproductive technologies and procreation.

3.7 Transformations in the Rationalities Governing the Policy Issue of Access

The chaotic parliamentary processes in 1996, along with a lack of party politics, have been put forward as explanations for the amendment of restricted access which 'almost appear accidental' (Albæk et al., 2012, p. 154). When examining the political process in 1996, I additionally point to the fact that the strong focus on controlling the possible implications of the emerging technological possibil-ities, brought with it a more or less intentional attempt to reinforce and reassert well-known and established family practises. In addition to delineating the core element of strategic framing, the comparative analysis also points to changes in the 'field of possibilities' (Foucault, 1983, p. 221) with regard to the discursively understanding of ART and family formation as implicitly underpinning the changes in policy positions. Whether or not ARTs propagate a social, legal, cultural, biological, genetic or technological understanding of parenthood is an ongoing discussion, and the intertwinement of shifting socio-historical pre-conditions and increasing technological possibilities in understanding family transformations is complex and not easily delineated. The increasing acceptance and routinization of reproductive technologies in a Danish context (Andersen et al., 2012) and in other Western societies (Franklin, 2008) have for instance – along with their corresponding family transformations – been interpreted in terms of a growing biomedical production (Cooper and Waldby, 2014, p. 61).

In the following section, I limit the analysis to the argument that the changing understandings of family practices and reproductive technology influenced the rationalities governing the policy issue of access, and that these changes are also reflected in the biopolitical understandings of the nature–culture distinction. Whereas Rose sees a dissolution of this distinction, in this analysis, the 'nature–culture' boundary is not dissolved but has merely been reconfigured in the years intervening between the early and late debates. This accentuates the idea of this boundary being continuously fluid and precarious. Still, the distinction is clearly expressed in the later debate, reflecting a technocentric biopolitics dealing with the advantages and disadvantages in the regulation of new biotechnology and the question of where to (re)establish the boundary. At the same time, the unstable boundary between nature and culture and between life and politics shows that life cannot only be considered a subject to political (intentional) actions and regula-tions but that it touches upon the foundational part of politics (Foucault, 1994, pp. 147ff; Lemke, 2009). Consequently, nature is not to be considered apart from politics and 'biology cannot be separated from political and moral questions' as Rose demonstrates (Lemke, 2009, p. 117).

Additionally, the new forms of moral (self-) governing and subjectification processes included in the ethopolitics concept are central features in the approach summarized within the culture frame. Understandings inherent to this frame include single and lesbian women being assigned with 'the rights to make life' to a greater extent, in relation to assisted reproduction for instance. This 'self-determination' constitutes a central feature of current biopolitics as well as notions of autonomy, rationality and choice (Lemke, 2009, p. 107; Memmi, 2003; Rose, 2007). Rose furthermore adds that whereas discipline normalizes, ethopo-litics focuses on self-actualizing (Rose, 2007, p. 18). Arguments posed within the culture frame reflect that single and lesbian women should increasingly be able to control and decide over their own 'reproductive conduct'. Moreover, they are positioned as reflexive individuals capable of rational behaviour. The fact that single and lesbian women in the later debate are portrayed as parents who are fully qualified to raise a child, accentuates the features of ethopolitics regarding 'self-determination' and 'the right to choose'. Still, single and lesbian women are governed according to current norms and values, but they are less reflected by traditional ideals highlighting biological notions vis-à-vis the nuclear family. Instead of drawing on techniques of discipline as the basis for regulation, this governmental approach broadens the foundation for normalization by operating with a more inclusive perception of family constellations. Despite efforts from the adherents of the nature frame to re-establish the increasingly fluid boundary between nature and culture by reinforcing nuclear family ideals, the analysis has shown that social changes have taken place towards a reframing of the issue of the rights of single and lesbian women to access reproductive technologies.

Overall, the analysis has shown that two main changes have taken place between the early and late debates: First, 'new family' formations such as solo mother families are increasingly accepted and second, there is a notable difference in the representation of ARTs which indicates that these technologies have been normalized to some extent. Furthermore, the analysis has also shown that these social changes can be seen as reflecting new biopolitical understandings. As Rose has argued, contemporary biopolitics has led more broadly to new regulation, risks and subjectivities. When comparing the two debates, we see the mobilization of the perspective of resistance has entailed a shift in power in how social meaning is constructed. The emerging rationality or 'style of thought' (Rose et al., 2006, p. 84) represented within this culture frame epitomizes a different kind of logic for how single and lesbian women should be governed within this area of ARTs. This emerging rationality also affects how single and lesbian women are discursively constructed in the debates, and this entails new forms of subjectivities being produced.

In short, these emerging understandings of procreation and family structures, to a greater extent, enable the construction of single and lesbian mothers as 'normal', 'good' and qualified parents that are to be included in a broader cate- gorization of our 'natural practices'. Regarding to the third element of risk, Rose has primarily emphasized genetic risks (Rose, 2007) whereas this analysis mainly considers the technological risks of ARTs. In considering the remarkable differ- ences between the ways in which the risks of these technologies are represented in the 1990s and 2000s respectively, the proliferation of ARTs could very well indicate that this development has affected the rise of pluralistic family under- standings and helped pave the way for a broader definition of what constitutes the 'natural order of life'. However, the policy controversy between the two main frames illustrates that the ideology of the biological nuclear family still constitutes a main narrative which marked the later debate. Nonetheless, new understandings of ARTs and family formation seem to be materializing, as the production of MAR legislation – also in relation to newer legislative additions such as double donation – seems to indicate a slowly growing acceptance of 'new families'.

Chapter 4

Revising Life Biographies: A Choice by Design and Not by Chance

This chapter explores how single women biographically and narratively account for their decision to embark upon solo motherhood. By asking how we are to understand this choice in a broader life story perspective and within the socio-cultural context in which the decision is made, this chapter shows how the women make sense of their choice and how dominating sociocultural narratives are adopted and challenged in the process. Drawing on findings from the biographical narrative interviews and on theoretical conceptualizations on life course and individualization, it explores the relations between the personal and the social and between the private and political from the individual point of view.

> We are in the middle of our stories and cannot be sure how they will end; we are constantly having to revise the plot as new events are added to our lives. Self, then, is not a static thing or a substance, but a configuring of personal events into an historical unity which includes not only what one has been but also anticipations of what one will be.
> —Polkinghorne (1988, p. 150)

While we are continually in a process of becoming, and the life story narratives we tell are situated in the present, they are always shaped by reconstructions of the past and anticipations of the future (Polkinghorne, 1988). This chapter details the interlinkages between past experiences, present actions and future anticipations of motherhood to gain insight into the motivations, biographical particulars and cultural settings that shape the decision to form a solo mother family.

In keeping with general findings on the driving forces which motivate people to pursue solo motherhood, the women interviewed would all have preferred to have a child within a relationship, and it has not been their intention to deselect a partner and/or father. The choice to embark upon solo motherhood is instead to be seen as a choice made due to a limited prospect of finding a suitable partner with whom to have a child. Studies within this field suggest that the limited prospect of becoming a mother within a relationship is related to considerations around

Lived Realities of Solo Motherhood, Donor Conception
and Medically Assisted Reproduction, 77–104
Copyright © 2021 Tine Ravn
Published under exclusive licence by Emerald Publishing Limited
doi:10.1108/978-1-83909-115-520211006

increasing age and fertility decline (see Bock, 2000; Golombok, 2015; Golombok et al., 2020; Graham, 2013). While this is also a general finding in this study, more than a third of the interviewees are in the beginning of their thirties when they initiate treatment. In contrast to most studies which show that women tend to be in their late thirties or early forties when embarking upon or becoming solo mothers (Bock, 2000; Golombok, 2015; Graham and Braverman, 2012; Grill, 2005; Jadva et al., 2009a; Mannis, 1999), this chapter will also explore the extent to which this diversity in age influences the women's decision-making process in terms of motivating factors. In this regard, the age aspect also raises the question of whether younger women contemplating solo motherhood are subjected to different normative reactions from their surroundings than women in their late thirties and early forties.

Graham (2013, p. 62) finds that 'solo motherhood is a "choice" borne out of constraint, one that is viewed with much ambivalence and anxiety regarding its acceptability and morality'. For the women in this study, the choice to pursue solo motherhood is also very much a moral decision and characterized with ambiguity, but rather than being framed as a 'no choice' narrative, it is discursively constructed as a narrative of 'best choice' (Graham and Ravn, 2016). This has implications for how the choice of solo motherhood is perceived; for how contradictions between real and ideal is narratively constructed and consequently for how agency is enacted and subject positions adopted. Studies have generally shown that the decision to embark upon solo motherhood is not taken lightly or 'overnight' but have matured over time. In this process, the anticipations of motherhood remain a decisive impetus.

4.1 Three Biographical Narratives on Contemplating Solo Motherhood

This section includes an analysis of three single biographical narratives that are centred on the decision to contemplate solo motherhood. They are included with the purpose to gain insight into the processes, motivations and biographical particulars that underlie this decision. The three narratives are exemplary in illustrating the main themes that emerge in the individual case plots. First, they portray the complex break between the real and ideal, and point to the diverse and shared strategies to handle such contradictions in the lived life as well as in the told story (the narrative). Second, they depict how the women's self-identification and – understandings change during the process of contemplating solo motherhood and how they position themselves according to greater cultural narratives on family formation. Third, in all of the 22 told stories, the interviewees include the transitional marker of not having found the right partner with whom to have a child. They have all carefully considered the option of embarking upon solo motherhood, but the three narratives included below illustrate that the process and ambivalence surrounding this decision turn out differently, for which diversity in age, in relationship history and treatment phase also play a part. Hence, the three single case analysis intend to illustrate the breadth of the narratives elicited and to act as a point of departure for the following analysis of main and shared themes across the complete sample of interviews.

4.1.1 Charlotte

Charlotte, 38, lives in Aarhus, the second largest city in Denmark, where she works as a physiotherapist. She has always wanted to start a family and have children, and early in her narrative she explicitly reflects on experiences that can explain her position as a single woman contemplating solo motherhood. She tells of an important turning point in the beginning of her thirties where she leaves a cohabiting partner with whom she planned to have a child. The issue of not having met the right partner with whom to start a family pose a recurring theme in Charlotte's account, and she tells of former relationships that have not worked out or where the partner has not been interested in having more children. In fact, before starting treatment at the age of 38, she ends a relationship because her partner did not want more children and she could not imagine a life without having children of her own. They have remained friends but both could not picture themselves in a constellation where they remained in a relationship while she attempted to get pregnant trough donor conception. At the time of the interview, Charlotte has undergone a first round of unsuccessful donor insemination. Due to her age and the tests she underwent, she was referred directly for IVF treatment, but was excluded for treatment the first time around and was instead offered a round of donor insemination.[1] She is now waiting to be able to sign up for IVF treatment again and also faces a change of donor, since her first choice of donor is no longer available.

The contemplation of solo motherhood has been in Charlotte's mind since her early thirties and since she ended the relationship with the former partner mentioned above. She had a single friend at the time who considered the possibility of having a donor-conceived child, and Charlotte became aware of this option through her. Charlotte was referred for treatment by her general practitioner at the age of 36 but postponed treatment due to her starting a new relationship. The hope of having a child within a relationship and her wish to secure a financial and permanent position as a physiotherapist have postponed her decision to go it alone but her increasing age and concerns about fertility decline have now motivated her to initiate treatment. She describes this trajectory as a 'major transformation process' and the plot line that structures her narrative account is one of development and progression in terms of making sense of her choice of departing from the type of family life she previously had imagined for herself. As she narrates:

> Because this is so huge, this longing, and for me it's not, how should I say it…for me a family doesn't have to consist of a mother, a father and children. Well, I want to…I've also accepted in myself that there are lots of different family forms, so in that way it's become the right choice for me. And the thought that I've made a decision to do this now, has also been a thought that's matured in my mind, so now it just feels completely right that it's something that I'm going to do myself. Because for me now, it's also that

---

[1] In the Danish public fertility clinics, you can be dismissed twice when signing up for IVF treatment due to daily capacity limitations.

I either do this alone, or I'm not going to have this child, because I can't wait any longer. And it feels right, because that's what I want. And I've even been to a psychologist a few times, and this is going to sound totally therapy-like, it's not, but to kind of let go of this dream of the traditional nuclear family – and that has been a loss for me – and to say, yes, but that's not what you should focus on now, to become this, because this is what I want. She also really helped me with prioritising, and what I should be focusing on, and what I want, and that I can't ride on more than one horse at a time, I need to make a choice.

Charlotte's narrative illustrates that the decision to parent alone and to depart from her wish to have a child within the two-parent family structure has not been taken lightly or overnight. It has been a process of coming to terms of that which could have been and grief regarding the fact that this has not and probably cannot be realized within the structures she has always considered to be ideal. As she states:

Because at the start, it was also a battle against myself, like I was thinking, "God, it was never this that I imagined". If you'd asked me 20 years ago, then I would have had a family and two kids right now. So there have been lots of processes in my own mind that needed to change.

Charlotte's biographical narrative most clearly illustrates that the ideal versus real in terms of life plans that can be realized, constitute both a process of applying meaning to past experiences and choices, as well as of negotiation and normalization. In Charlotte's case, she actively makes a difficult choice to find new biographical solutions as a strategy to align her life situation with what she finds to be ideal. She argues that time will soon run out in terms of being able to become pregnant, whereas this is not the case with meeting a future partner that may become a social father for her child. In her decision-making process, she has also challenged her own previous ideals – and the traditional family values with which she has been raised – with the idea that family life can take on other shapes than the traditional heterosexual nuclear one, and she argues that the Danish society in general is characterized by a rich variety in family constellations. For instance, she has been in relationships with men who already have children and she argues that a similar construction will be the case if she is the one who brings a donor-conceived child into the relationship. Despite aligning her current choices as close as possible to her initial dreams and wishes, Charlotte repeatedly points to the transformative character of the ideal. Hence, her choice of opting for solo motherhood is not to be perceived as plan A or as a 'second best'. In the beginning of her narrative she explicitly states that:

Now, this sounds like it's some sort of 'second best', but it's really not for me, not anymore. Well, I've gotten older and this hope for, this desire to find a man, it might have sort of faded, because I've also been thinking, "I'm not going to make it, and then I'm not going to be able to have this child.

At the end of the interview, she returns to this recurring plot by saying;

I hope that throughout this interview, because I've been referring to this thing about not having found this man, and it's not like, it's not, again, like some kind of emergency solution, it's not second best, it's an active choice that I've made.

When asked at the end of the interview whether she has any concluding thoughts or comments she once again states that:

I've had some other expectations, hopes, dreams, both earlier and later on. But I really do hope that people understand that this is really my number one choice right now and that's it's not just for a lack of a better alternative." [...]. It's not because I don't want to start a family, but I'm just maybe doing things in a different order. Because I don't, well, my biological clock is about to run out, so I have to, or I want to have a child, and that's what I'm acting on right now. So I can meet the man later. After all, there's no clock ticking on that one, hopefully...

To Charlotte, solo motherhood may not be her initial plan A but it is not her plan B or a 'second best', either. Rather, the field of possibilities has changed, as have her current circumstances, and within this context, donor conception then becomes the new ideal in terms of the options available. Charlotte is revising her biography accordingly and it is important to her that this revision and adaptation is represented as an act of agency. Through the 'voice' of an acquaintance who asks Charlotte whether she 'has given up', Charlotte narratively positions herself. The use of other 'voices' in a life story interview serves the objective of categorization and negotiating meaning with the greater aim of self-identification (Horsdal, 2012, p. 94). Charlotte states that the idea of 'giving up' was not part of her mindset and her self-understanding; rather, she considers her decision to pursue solo motherhood as a strong one and one by which she wholeheartedly acts on her great desire to become a mother. In general, she has received a lot of support from her closest network and she explains that this has also had a decisive impact on her decision.

While the means of becoming a mother has changed, the end goal of having an own child has not. The desire to become a mother runs as a plot line around which Charlotte's narrative unfolds and this motivation interconnects the dimensions of past, present and future in her account; she is at a point in her decision-making process at which she has reworked and revised her ideals of family life. She is currently still in the process of undergoing fertility treatment and at a point at which her anticipation of becoming a mother has not yet been realized. In this sense, becoming a mother remains an important factor in her life plans and the vision of becoming a mother in the future forms an important part of the way she constructs her identity.

> The thing that psychologically...or that makes me vulnerable, is the thought that it might not happen. There's no guarantee. If only you could know that it was going to happen. It would just be a question of whether it would take a year, or two or three, but I could be certain that out there in the future, it would happen for me. But you don't know that, and then there's something somewhere in me that starts to think, "how is your life going to be if you don't have kids?" Because so much of my life is based on the idea that I'll be a mother in the future. Or not based on, but the way I think about the future. And THAT is vulnerable. And it's a real rollercoaster when I think, 'God, what then?'.

The vulnerable state of not knowing whether she will be able to fulfil her wish to become a mother and the insecurity of potentially having to re-examine her life and consequently redefine her sense of self, adds to the 'emotional rollercoaster' (Thompson, 2005, p. 93) that defines Charlotte's process of undergoing fertility treatment. This is also connected to her explicit reference to not being comfortable considering alternative ways of becoming a mother, through egg donation or adoption for instance, because she needs to believe that her current treatment process will be successful.

4.1.2 Mette

Mette, 39, holds a leading position in a teaching institution. She lives in Northern Jutland, close to her parents and sister. She is trained as a teacher and has worked as a primary school teacher for a number of years at various public schools. Being a teacher, she recurrently experienced dissatisfaction with her job and after two periods of sick leave due to stress, she decides to quit her job and figure out what she wants to do with her professional life. This event marks the first greater turning point in her narrative account. As an 'existential act' (Denzin, 1989, p. 71), Mette tells about this job transition as a threshold to begin a new but related professional career, and she highlights the positive effects of this experience as one that led her to the job she now holds and with which she is very satisfied. When asked to tell her life story from when she finished lower secondary school, it is perhaps not surprising that she opens her story with educational/ professional achievements and developments as part of a chronologically ordered telling. Moreover, life story narratives are often structured around turning points that indicate change and biographical revisions (Horsdal, 2012). This is also the case in Mette's account but the revision is not externally driven; she is the one who takes control to bring about change. She describes this turning point in a straight-forward way and as a matter of fact but narratively, she implicitly positions herself as a strong and independent woman, who actively manages difficult experiences in order to achieve positive change. Later in her narrative account, she also describes herself as a person whose nature it is to make a decision and carry it out in a determined manner.

This positioning counterbalances the doubt that characterizes her private situation and that comes across as a struggle between accepting external factors in the shape of 'fate' and actively counteracting her current situation by making use of the options available. In fact, she continues her story with the plot that comes to structure her entire narrative account; the decision to contemplate solo motherhood and the ambivalence that surrounds this choice.

Mette has always had an enormous wish to start a family but has never met a man with whom she could do so. She has never been in a long-term relationship and throughout her thirties she continues to hope that she will meet a partner, and this hope prevents her from pursuing solo motherhood. She tells of years of doubt, of knowing about the possibility of having a donor-conceived child but she describes how a dogged determination to go down this road seemed a bit 'consumeristic' and that it clashed with her view that the achievement of a loving relationship and having children should be seen as a gift and approached in a humble fashion. Her strong wish for a child and her age are decisive factors for her starting treatment when at the age of 39. Support from her general practitioner and especially from her close network also helps her decision along. At the time of the interview, Mette has been through three rounds of unsuccessful donor inseminations (IUI-D). From the first referral to treatment, and between treatments, she has felt it necessary to take smaller breaks in order to feel that she is fully onboard each time. She has decided to continue with IUI treatment but is facing a change of donor in order to increase the success rate, and is undecided on whether to continue with an identity-release donor (see also Chapter 7). The choice of donor constitutes a moral decision as does the decision to contemplate solo motherhood:

> I'm choosing to do this alone, and I think I can stand up for that and explain to a future child why I've made that choice. And there isn't, yeah, I don't think there's a right and a wrong. It's about how I feel about it and that I can defend it. But that's what I'm thinking about a lot right now. And also about when I want to, again, well, I feel like I can really, deep in myself, I'm not in any doubt that this is something that I want, but what I think is really difficult, is that I really have a great life. It's not like I feel like I need a child to fulfil something. Like not at all. And I still have this discussion, "yeah but Mette, you've got this great life, with lots of opportunities and freedom". It's a major crossroad for me, about what direction my life should take. That's something I'm still fighting with, and I think that's also why there have been long breaks in between my attempts, because I really need to make sure I'm on-board. And of course I also think about whether I can give this child what it needs. Will it be too difficult to be a single mother, and well, there are a huge number of thoughts in that.

The quotation above reveals the complexity and ambiguity inherent in Mette's narrative. On the one hand, she expresses confidence in making the choice to contemplate solo motherhood and she feels comfortable in rationalizing her decision. On the other hand, she invokes the strong metaphor of finding herself at a crossroad in her life, being unsure which road to take next. She very much wants to experience motherhood, and she believes she has a lot to offer to a child. With the metaphor of 'a ticking clock' she also cannot rely on the idea of meeting a man because – not knowing when or if he will come along – it will probably be 'too late' to have a child. At the same time, she morally questions the decision to have a donor-conceived child who will grow up not knowing its biological father. In her narrative, she also states that she has a good life and that in a somewhat religious and superstitious way, is able to believe that her life has turned out the way it has for a reason. Again, we see a strong 'clash of values' (Horsdal, 2012, p. 96) in her narrative between accepting 'fate' and the life chances given on the one hand, and taking matters into her own hands in actively making life plans that involve becoming a solo mother on the other. To Mette, the ambivalence defining her meaning-making process is also characterized by a schism between science and religious belief and between natural and not natural:

> I'm a religious person in many ways, and as I said before, well, I've always thought that - both finding love and having children – I've always had this sense of humility about it, that it's something that will happen in my life if it's meant to be. So for that reason it's been challenging for me to make a decision and say, yes but now I'm going to take advantage of science and the opportunities it provides, so that I can fulfil a huge wish.

To Mette, it is not morally wrong to make use of the possibilities given by reproductive technology, but the theme of 'naturalness' intersects with navigating between 'fate' and 'choice'. She states that the decision to have a child comes more 'natural' in a relationship, and in terms of treatment, the issue of staying close to the 'natural' process of reproduction with the use of as few 'remedies' as possible, also proves important to her:

> Well I think the reason I don't, or about thinking about it too much, is about wanting to take things one step at a time, and to say that now, this is where I am and there's not much point in thinking about all kinds of other things [...] I'm not sure either that I'll continue, if it doesn't work with this...how should I say it... slightly more natural attempt. I'm not sure that I have enough courage to go through all kind of other things. I don't think so actually. Then I think I would just accept it, and say, ok, so it wasn't meant to be [...] Maybe I don't want it SO much that I'm prepared to go through all kinds of things with my body, and maybe have lots of hormones and feel strange because of it – I don't have the courage for that. I'm pretty clear about that,

right now in any case. But of course that could change pretty quickly if this doesn't work, because if the desire is still really strong, then I'll probably be willing to try anything.

Mette describes the process of fertility treatment in a way that comes to define many of the life story narratives in this study: the initial wish to stay as close to the natural process as possible; the reluctance to plan treatment ahead out of fear that the current round of treatment will not be successful, and the issue of redefining one's boundaries for treatment procedures during the process. This issue will be treated separately in the following chapter, but Mette's description clearly illustrates the process of rationalization that serves to give meaning to the outcome both of her 'emotional rollercoaster' (Thompson, 2005, p. 93) decision-making process and the success of her treatment procedure, as a way of arguing that things happen for a reason regardless of the outcome. As she also states in the first part of her narration: 'I think it's really kind of up and down in this process'.

As with the clash of values mentioned above, Mette also tells how she has altered her 'conservative' ideal of the nuclear family to include other types of families as well, and that in forming a solo mother family, she will be able to offer a child other types of relationships. While Mette narrates her story in a difficult life passage that is marked by ambivalence, her account is also characterized by her reworking and redefining some of her previous ideals and beliefs. She expresses the main argument of her narrative in the following way: 'I just think that the urge is so strong, that I have to compromise on the values I have and have had'. The break between real and ideal and the ambivalence this break carries with it, comes across most clearly and forcefully in Mette's narrative, although this break constitutes a general theme across the collective life story narratives.

Despite the clash of values expressed in Mette's account, her narrative also reveals temporal change in her reworking of her notions of the ideal versus real, and the decision to start fertility treatment comes across as a transformatory experience and an important turning point that may lead to fulfilling the ideal of starting a family of her own, despite compromising other ideals. At the end of her narrative she makes it clear that she chooses to redirect her biography by claiming agency and not leaving her life trajectory up to 'fate' alone. In this regard she constructs and sustains her self-understanding as a person who purposefully makes and carries out strong decisions:

> I try to always choose to see the strong aspects to it, to kind of focus on the fact that it is pretty brave to dare to launch into a project like this alone. And it shows that you have surplus resources, strength and a belief that you can do it [...] It's a completely conscious, goal-focused decision. It's important for me to stand firm on that. And it's also important for me, the thing that, as I also said earlier, I'm not doing it because there's something I need to fulfil in my life. You know, that I'm lonely or lacking content in my life, that's really important for me

because that's way too much of a burden to put on a child, to have to fulfil that kind of role. So it's because I want to, and because I want it. I have a good life, but I think it would be even better if I was allowed to become a mother and have a child to take care of.

4.1.3 Sarah

Sarah, 32, is a mother of a four-year-old donor-conceived child, and at the time of the interview, she is pregnant with her second child, also conceived through donor insemination (IUI-D). She lives in a smaller city north of Copenhagen, close to her nearest family and friends. She is trained and works as a pedagogue. Her parents divorced when Sarah was eight years old and she and her sister continued to live with their mother. She describes herself as a 'tomboy' and she explains that – apart from a number of male acquaintances – she has not been in a long-term relationship and that she has always thrived being on her own. She has always wanted to have children and she imagined that she would become a mother by the age of 25. When she retrospectively reports this period in her life, she describes a frustration of not being at the point in her life that she initially imagined herself to be. At that time she considers contemplating solo motherhood at the age of 30 if she still has not met a partner with whom to have a child. In her narrative account she refers to a greater turning point in her life at the age of 27:

> When I turned 27, I thought "Why should I wait for him, when I'm so comfortable being on my own?" So then I spent some time thinking about that. And I was thinking so intensively for a couple of months, and then went to a journal conversation and consciously planned that it should be in half a year, so I could have a good amount of time to get used to it and find out, is this what I want. And I actually experienced that from the moment I took the decision, that I didn't have the scruples either about my age or where I was in my life, and that my winter depression disappeared completely automatically, and I haven't had it since. And I felt like, all of a sudden, from thinking that I was going in one direction in my life, that I was going in another, but that it was the right direction for me.

Sarah invokes the metaphor of taking the right route in life to describe her decision to contemplate solo motherhood. As a turning point, it can be characterized as a form of epiphany that Denzin denotes the 'major event' which 'alter[s] the fundamental meaning structures in a person's life' (Denzin, 1989, pp. 70–71). In Sarah's narrative, this decision represents a positive resolution to a personal conflict. The plot twist of redirecting her biography from the expected trajectory in taking the route 'less travelled by' (Frost, 1949, p. 131) is described as a meaningful and transformatory experience. In the few words of 'why wait' lie a break with the 'normal' biography and its more standardized norms for life course structuring. In Sarah's case, it is not age as a single parameter but her age combined with taking a less standardized route to motherhood that signals a break with the ideal. The first time she started IUI-treatment and went for a record consultation, she experienced that her choice to become a solo mother was questioned:

> It was a special experience because I experienced some prejudice, or that I wasn't met with the same support because I was too young. She asked, 'You're very young?'. I was 27 at the time, and how I should maybe find a man, and had I thought it through properly, and it's a big job. I felt like people were talking down to me a little bit. And I don't think it was her intention, but my experience was that when you've heard about the others, like she said, then I was young in comparison, and also when I've read about it sometimes, you hear that when you choose to be a solo mother, it's because you haven't found the one man in your life, and she thought that it was very early for me to give up, like you need to have struggled with it for many years and then because you couldn't find happiness in the way you would most like to, then you could choose this as plan B. And where I'd arrived at in my realization was that this was my plan A. It wasn't going to be my plan B, so yeah, it was a bit of a special experience. But I stood my ground anyway. Yes.

Sarah did not experience being asked similar questions when she initiated treatment for the purpose of becoming pregnant with her second child. In general, it seems as if the choice of contemplating solo motherhood is more acceptable from a societal perspective if the decision is made due to 'time running out' and it being the last option for having a child of one's own. Sarah's narrative then, points not only to societal expectations around the forming of families in general, but also expectations around the (last call) motivations for forming solo mother families. The much-applied terminology of plan a and b is also invoked by Sarah to stress that her decision to parent alone is not a 'second best' option but her preferred choice.

In this regard, she also narrates that

> I've never – and this is where I think my [parents'] divorce maybe plays a role - I've never really believed in myself in a relationship, where we should be together forever. I couldn't bear the thought of sharing my children with a man that I couldn't make it work with. I don't think I could do that. And I hold relationships in really high regard, and I think it's fantastic when my girlfriends live in these relationships and I'm so happy for them, but at the same time, I also thrive really well when it's just me and my daughter.

Sarah revisits the theme of her parent's divorce several times in her narrative account to express how she believes this event has influenced her and her choice to form a solo mother family. Living with her sister and mother after her parent's divorce has also influenced her choice in the sense that her own positive experience with this particular family constellation has given her a belief in the quality of solo mother families. She also restates how she thrives being alone with her daughter, and says later in the interview that one advantage of the solo mother family form is never having to share her child with a former partner, and that her daughter will never be a child of divorced parents and 'be caught between a rock and a hard place'.

In making the choice to contemplate solo motherhood, from which it follows that her children will not have a biogenetic father present in their lives, it has been important for Sarah that her children are able to access information about their paternal biogenetic inheritance when they reach adulthood. At the time she undergoes treatment for her first child, the option of using an identity-release donor was only available in midwife-run (non-doctor) clinics (see also Chapter 7), and Sarah chooses to pay for treatment herself in such a clinic. She also reserved 10 portions of donor sperm (straws) from the same donor, because she knew that she would like to have another child and would like them to be biogenetically related. Regarding the latter, she wanted to provide them with the same set of options, primarily in terms of being able to contact and potentially meet the donor. Sarah postponed having a second child until she felt her daughter was old enough (she will be five-year-old when she becomes a big sister) and until she had secured a permanent job. She did not want her daughter to be an only child, but to have a sibling. As she states,

> Also because I've chosen to bring her into the world without a father, and I would like her to be able to share it with someone, just like I shared the divorce with my sister, you know to have that in common. That was really important for me.

Sarah's narrative is primarily ordered around the plot line of being a 'mother with a capital M'; of the ways in which she prioritizes her daughter in their daily life and how being a mother acts to forge identity and create meaning in Sarah's life.

> I'm a mother now and I will be for the rest of my life, but right you are that in a different way when you have small children, and then the time where I can develop myself, that comes later. But that means a lot to me and I love that role, well it's a huge part of me. Well, the largest part, I identify with that, and I'm really like, I enjoy going around with my daughter and just being us.

Throughout her narrative, Sarah talks about experiences and events that support the plot of prioritizing her daughter and creating a well-functioning everyday life for them. Such events included and include practical arrangements such as moving closer to her family, reducing work hours, postponing career ambitions and scaling down participation in various social events. She was also involved in a part-time relationship for a while, but ended the relationship due to the realization that such an arrangement does not work optimally for her when concurrently having small children.

In addition to the considerations described above regarding Sarah's decision-making process, she also talks about enormous support from her closest network and of having been raised in a way that has fostered 'a pretty strong self-esteem around daring to be who I am'. When asked whether any societal conditions have influenced her decision to form a solo mother family, she says,

> The fact that more and more people are getting divorced and there are more and more that are living alone, and that means that you don't stand out so much, I think of course that's definitely been significant. I think it's been significant that even back then, I can remember reading about families where they lived apart, but were still a family, and I got quite inspired by that, I thought it was interesting in relation to the idea that I thrive well just being myself. And that there are lots of people that actively choose to be alone. If I'd been young in the 80s, I'm not sure I would have done it. So, anyway, there had to be some people to tread the path before you dare to do it yourself. But at the same time, I was the first one in my network to do it. But I also have a network that means that I've never been in any doubt, where it doesn't matter that you do things a little alternatively or are different. So yeah.

The passage above points to a number of sociocultural issues that broadly characterize the narrative accounts in this study; general changes in family demographics have broadened the normative span for cultural narratives on doing family, akin to increasing the important element of being able to identify with others when reworking the still dominant cultural narrative of the two-parent family model. Sarah's statement illustrates the double construction of enacting agency in choosing a road 'less travelled by' (Frost, 1949, p. 131) but one than nonetheless has been carved out by others and structurally made possible to travel.

4.2 Motivating the Decision – A Choice by Design and Not by Chance

What can be said about single women pursuing solo motherhood? Do they share a number of characteristics other than the desire to have a child and a wish to experience motherhood? Are they the epitome of their negative and stereotypical portrayal; selfish career women who are particularly choosy when it comes to choice of partner or who wish to deselect men altogether? Although relatively little research exists on choice mother characteristics (Golombok, 2015), the

Danish and international studies within the area cannot confirm this negative collective portrait. The Danish survey study on single mothers embarking upon solo motherhood for example, found no 'significant differences [...] regarding socio-demographic characteristics, previous long-term relationships, previous pregnancies or attitudes towards motherhood' (Salomon et al., 2015, p. 473) apart from the fact that they were 3.5 years older on average than the comparison group of cohabiting women. The socio-demographic attributes characterizing this study's cross section of single women is described in Appendix 1, and while they added to the picture of single women being professional and financially secure, they also showed diversity in terms of age, geographical location, and civil status (previous marriages, existing children).

In a humorous tone, Anne depicts the gap between her own initial pre-sumptions about single mothers by choice and the women she subsequently became acquainted with:

> When I was asked if I would be a part of this networking group for solo mothers, I thought, yeeaah, but who are these other girls? They're guaranteed to all be like lesbian manhaters. There won't be anyone like me, completely normal, that look normal, have a normal job and who think more or less normally. And then I met ten other girls that were just like me. They weren't ugly, or lesbians, or manhaters, they didn't have anything totally traumatic in their baggage, just completely normal girls. [...] I don't think it's for everyone, if I had to try to find something that is common among the people I know who are doing this, it's people that are goal-oriented, dynamic, that have the courage to do something, kind of open to different ways of thinking. But other than that, we're quite normal. I think it's that thing of maybe being curious or open to other alternatives.
> –Anne (pharmaconomist, in treatment with IVF)

In addition to common socio-economic attributes, Anne points to a shared sentiment of drive and determination as well as openness to deviate from more well-travelled life trajectories. However, can such sentiments and life choices be traced in the plot lines of the women's biographical narratives?

4.2.1 Independence and Nurture: Narrative Themes and Life Story Plots

While the introductory narratives only represent a section of the told stories of the interviewees, they clearly illustrate individual complexity regarding biographical particularities, motivations and rationales. However, when comparing the lived experiences emphasized in the plot story of the women's biographical narratives, shared themes and common plots can be traced. In general, the theme of *independence and nurture* interweaves understandings of self with the sequence of biographical experiences: Common plots include events such as travels and studies abroad in early youth, national relocations due to studies and work opportunities in youth and adulthood. Some tell of becoming adults fairly early, which forges independence from a young age, of taking the role of nurturer in sibling relations or among friends. For many, the element of nurture intersects with the choice of occupation, of internal and external self-identification of being great with children, and many tell of having close relations to nieces and nephews.

The plots also trace an educational and professional drive to follow new and sometimes unexpected career choices; not to prioritize career over having children but merely as an integration of the connection between work and family life that has come to define the female 'normal biography' in Danish society. Most know from early youth that they would like to become mothers, and while they express openness towards alternative ways of living and forming family, they imagine for themselves that they will raise their children within the more traditional family setting. Throughout their twenties and thirties, typical turning points include the ending of short or long-term relationships and increasing concerns about fertility decline. The limited prospect of finding a partner marks a process of rethinking and reworking their own family ideals and negotiating a departure from them. For most, the realization that they need to prioritize a child over a partner if they are to become mothers emerges gradually, although some more prospectively integrate the possibility of embarking upon solo motherhood into their biographical project with the typical statement 'if I have not met a partner at the age of x, then I will go it alone'. The position of motherhood remains a strong identifier throughout the biographical narratives and appears impervious to transcendence. This continuous identification is projected into future visions of motherhood, and current self-understandings and life plans are transformed accordingly.

4.2.2 Motivations and Justifications for Embarking upon Solo Motherhood

Why do single women choose to pursue solo motherhood? In keeping with the general findings within the area, single women make the decision to embark upon solo motherhood because they have not found the right partner with whom to have a child as a result of various factors, and their great desire to experience motherhood and concerns about increasing age and fertility decline motivate them to initiate treatment before it is 'too late' for them to have a child of their own. When talking about the decision-making process, these motivational factors also emerge from the women's life story narratives in this study. Like Charlotte, many mention anticipations for the future that clearly include visions of motherhood, and they identify themselves by this self-projection. Becoming mothers is seen as a key element in their biography, akin to creating a family within the more traditional setting. If they are to succeed with both, they need to rework the order of the biographical elements, and therefore many state that a child needs to come first and then a partner may follow later on. The plot twist is a strategy to minimize the tension between the real and the ideal, to mend 'biographical discontinuity' (Tjørnhøj-Thomsen, 2003, p. 64), and the decision is primarily justified by a biological and 'naturalized' need to experience motherhood (cf. Chapter 6).

In this regard, many explicitly state that they believe they will be 'good mothers' who will have a lot to offer a child. Many also use the 'voices' of others in their narration to substantiate this construction by referencing typical statements such as 'if you shouldn't do it, who should?' to stress and manage the impression (Goffman, 1992) that just as much as others, they consider themselves to be qualified and resourceful women who will be able to provide very well for their children, and as the plot in Sarah's narrative clearly illustrates, committed to put the child's need above their own. In echoing the findings from Graham (2013, p. 113) that single women embarking upon solo motherhood 'place the welfare of their imagined child at the forefront of their decision-making', the women in this study have been through a process of careful deliberations in which they have 'tried to think through every possibly scenario' as Mille states (insurance consultant, daughter age 2 through IUI-D).

In addition to their route to motherhood through sperm donation being by design and not by chance, nothing is left to chance when planning for life as a solo mother. In securing the well-being of the child, two types of resources are emphasized: First, the ability to be a qualified parent as mentioned above, and to secure the psychological well-being of the child by being a loving, independent, strong parent who put the needs of the child first. In a similar manner to the findings in the study by Bock (2000), the interviewees stress the personal attributes of 'responsibility' and 'emotional maturity'. The latter comprises 'a sufficient degree of self-confidence, psychological health, and assertiveness. Part of this includes coming to terms with one's single status' (2000, p. 72). Like Charlotte, some explicitly tell of coming to terms with the grief of departing from the two-parent family form, but the decision-making process in general is characterized by working through the ambivalence of becoming the sole parent. Second are the material and social surroundings: It is important to provide a safe and stable environment for their children through the securing of a permanent job, and the provision of a suitable home and social network for themselves and their children, and the women have organized their lives accordingly as also reflected in the biographical narratives by Charlotte, Mette and Sarah above.

In addition to the 'biological need' as a justification to pursue solo motherhood, some also mention the cultural and social significance of having children; of seeing one's immediate circle of acquaintances forming partnerships and families and wanting to follow the same life phase trajectory that 'tie[s] motherhood to womanhood, parenthood to adulthood' (Hertz, 2006, p. 19, see Chapter 1 for a discussion of the sociocultural significance of children). Hence, the cultural narrative of perceiving motherhood and parenthood as 'an inevitable part of a woman's normal life course' (Sevón, 2005, p. 462) is also adopted by the interviewees and it provides grounds for justifying their decision. As evident from Sarah's narrative, and from the majority of life stories at large, the decision to take this particular route to parenthood is also motivated by the fact that Danish society comprises a profusion of different family forms. The greater acceptance of different family constructions and the possibility for the interviewees and their children to identify with others who live in single-parent and/or blended families etc. adds to the normalization of their choice. In this regard, being able to read, hear, network or meet others and gain more knowledge/share experience about solo motherhood and having a child through donor conception has also proven important to many.

In general, the decision to embark upon solo motherhood can be characterized as a process of deliberation and many have contemplated the decision for years. The pros and cons of embarking upon solo motherhood are carefully considered and friends, family, general practitioners, among others, are often consulted in the process. The following statement by Ditte characterizes the core moral dilemma in the process:

> Should I wait until I find a boyfriend, or find someone, or should I just throw myself into it? And I used a long time on that, at least a couple of years going back and forth, because I think it was a really, really difficult decision, not so much for myself or what it consists of practically, but more because my big dilemma was that you opt out of something on the child's behalf, and the child doesn't have a choice, and I think that's hard. But when the decision was made, well if, and then I've read a lot about it and that really helped me a lot.
>
> –Ditte, (lawyer, daughter age 1 via ICSI)

While the resources required and the practical consequences have been well-considered and organized and many have grieved over the loss of a partner with whom to start a family, it is primarily the loss of a father/second parent that causes the moral dilemma and the ambivalence experienced. Mirroring the negative public opinion on this issue, the women ask themselves if their choice is selfish and what the consequences for a child to be donor-conceived and to grow up without the presence of its biological father will be. To some extent, the dilemma regarding 'the need for a father' (Gamble, 2009) remains an integral part of making the choice and impossible to solve. The interviewees need to believe that it will not be detrimental for a child to grow up in a solo mother family without a father and they substantiate this with the strong belief that they will be able to give their children a happy childhood surrounded by other close social relations, including male role models, who will love and support the child. In addition, most hope and some plan more actively for a future partner who will be able to act as a social father/second partner for their child. Some use existing research on solo mother families and/or the lived experiences from other solo mother families as evidence that children generally thrive very well in solo mother families. The pluralization of today's family forms is again a typical way to rationalize that many children experiences different constellations of family formation and that their child will not be the only one among their peers not to be raised in the traditional nuclear family. Rationalizing the choice is also strongly connected to the choice of using donor insemination, and making the child's conception story into a narrative about positive choice and not about active deselection on the part of the biological father (for a detailed discussion on this issue see Chapter 6).

4.2.3 A 'Double Yoke of Responsibility': Biographical Experiences and Turning Points

For all interviewees, making the decision is a process of deliberation that has been shaped by a number of previous biographical experiences and turning points. For most, it is not a single event which acts as the triggering factor but instead is characterized by a complex set of contributory causes, as illustrated in the introductory narratives. For Charlotte, a triggering event is her leaving a partner who does not want more children, but as evident from her biographical narrative, other relationship experiences and fertility considerations play a significant part, too. For Sarah, the turning point and 'why wait epiphany' she experiences at the age of 27 constitutes a catalytic event but is based on former experiences of unsuccessful short-term relationships. This is also the case for Mette, although she realizes more gradually that she needs to begin fertility treatment if she is to become a mother. While the transitional marker of not having found the right partner is a common plot in the life stories, their relationship histories comprise different turning point types.

All women have previously been in relationships, and this is also in keeping with nurse and network coordinator Maria Salomon's assessment that the single women she meets at Rigshospitalet have all been active in terms of dating (Salomon, expert interview, see presentation, appendix 1). Broadly speaking, the women in this study fall in two main groups in terms of relationship history. One group of 10 interviewees – as in the case of Sarah and Mette – have generally experienced more short-terms relationships that have not involved living together with a partner. The other group of interviewees ($n = 12$) have generally been in a number of long-term relationships and these relationships along with their endings, generally play a more significant role in the plot lines of their life stories. On the whole, the ending of a long-term relationship also marks a more significant turning point that is of significant or decisive importance for the decision to embark upon solo motherhood for this group of interviewees.

Four of the women have previously been married, and two of these women have a child with their former husbands. A main motivation for them to initiate fertility treatment is a wish for another child and a younger sibling for their children. Anne divorced her husband at the age of 34, and after a period of dating without meeting a potential partner, she starts to contemplate solo motherhood. A catalytic event for Anne is when she finds out at the age of 37 that she has blocked fallopian tubes and that she needs IVF treatment to become pregnant. Her doctor advises her to start treatment right away with the words 'there is not a moment to lose' and Anne describes this as a 'wake up call' and a pivotal motivational factor to start treatment. At the age of 34, Karen Marie is ready, together with her husband, to initiate fertility treatment. Her husband has previously been diagnosed with cancer and has been through a course of illness. Before they begin fertility treatment, her husband starts to get ill again. His condition quickly deteriorates and after a few months he dies. Five years later, Karen Marie has not met a new partner with whom to have a child and after years of contemplation, she decides to go it alone. At the time of the interview, she is four months pregnant. In a similar manner to other interviewees, she brings up the issue of becoming single in one's thirties:

> I think I've been single in a period in my life that's really difficult to be single in, because none of my friends or girlfriends have been single, they've all been in the nesting phase and the career phase and all those things, and they've been either pregnant or had small children, so it wasn't like they could go out into town with her, the single friend every other weekend. So that period from 35 to 40, also because people generally have children later, so it is then that most people have kids, right?
>
> –Karen Marie (support worker, pregnant through IVF)

Despite the fact that the structuring of life courses has become less standardized over time, and a pluralization of life worlds' (Flick, 2009, p. 12), characterizes modern ways of living, 'normative life-events' such as specific age norms for starting a family still structure the 'normal biography' (Heinz and Krüger, 2001, pp. 37–38; Hoerning, 2001, p. 121). Many experience that it is more difficult to meet a partner in the later part of one's thirties since many have already established families in this phase of their life or have already ended their marriages/relationships again. Several women tell of meeting men who do not want children or men who already have children and do not want another child. In this regard, some of the interviewees explicitly state that it might be easier to meet a partner if they have a child themselves when they enter into a relationship, and that this would then resemble the more endemic blended family model. Their view on the blended family model clearly illustrates the changes in family demographics (described in Chapter 1) and the increasingly accepted 'recomposed' family formations as a result of divorce and remarriages/new partnerships. Giddens notion of 'pure relationships' – of relationships being formed (and ended) on the basis of emotional and reciprocal relations rather than on more practical and rational grounds (1991) – provides a suitable characterization of both the individual and collective cultural perceptions of forming the 'right' emotive relationships that are expressed in the women's narratives.

In general, their views depict the pluralization of actual lived family experience and illustrate the materialization and transformation of discursive and normative expectations – in this case of family practices – through which identities are constituted (Butler, 1993). In other words, the increasing normalization of blended families has expanded the possibilities for adopting new subject positions and for 'doing family' but this positioning also illustrates a need to enter into continuous dialogue with more established and accepted cultural models as a way of legitimizing and normalizing their choice to form solo mother families.

In several ways, the view on individual biographies expressed in the individualization theories represented by Beck/Beck-Gernsheim as well as Giddens illustrates this duality of pluralization and standardization. Making the choice to embark upon solo motherhood as a choice by design and not by chance bears witness to the increased possibilities provided within the 'elective biography' as one needed to be shaped and managed by the individual (Beck and Beck-Gernsheim, 2001). It reflects the idea that ourselves have increasingly become lifelong 'reflexive projects' through a narrative of self-identity that is continuously sustained and revised (Giddens, 1991). In epitomizing the mantra of the individualization thesis, Giddens states that 'in conditions of high modernity, we all not only follow lifestyles, but in an important sense are forced to do so – we have no choice but to choose' (1991, p. 81). With choice comes responsibility and we see a transformation from more predefined common destinies and fixed identities to an increased responsibility to construct one's own life trajectory (Giddens, 1991). The modern cultural narrative of individualization continues to be highly influential (Horsdal, 2012) and while enforcing states of reflexivity and personal responsibility due to the disembedding of tradition, it also carries with it new structures and insecurities, and the 'elective biography' is not just a matter of choice but also always a 'tightrope biography' that must be managed within new institutional boundaries (Beck and Beck-Gernsheim, 2001, p. 3). Hence, the 'pluralization of life worlds' (Flick, 2009, p. 12) broadly acts as a way to rationalize their choice while the tension between the reel and ideal are minimized through a general positioning against more establishing ways of 'doing family'. Overall, it seems as though the decision-making process is characterized by a '*double yoke of responsibility*' in having to manage the choices and insecurities ensuing from reflexive life projects and the break between destiny and choice (as exemplified by Mette's narrative), while also being subjugated to legitimizing the choice of solo motherhood and their own abilities as responsible mothers.

The break between real and ideal causes ambivalence and reveals a paradoxical feature of the 'choice' of embarking upon solo motherhood. This ambiguity primarily concerns 'the need for a father' (Gamble, 2009) as stated earlier and to the related wish of having children within the two-parent family constellation. However, based on the biographical findings, I argue that we must view the ideal vs. real as a process of mitigating the gap and constructing a 'narrative of best choice' (Graham and Ravn, 2016).

4.2.4 A 'Narrative of Best Choice': Mitigating the Real versus Ideal

The choice to contemplate solo motherhood is often described within the literature on single mothers by choice as an ambivalent choice: single women have been characterized as 'unwilling warriors' in the sense that they both promote solo motherhood whilst also holding on to 'hegemonic fantasies of normative family structures' (Bock, 2000, p. 70). The choice has also been described as a 'plan b' since solo motherhood is often not the initial planned route to family formation (Frederiksen et al., 2011); as 'less than ideal' (Zadeh et al., 2013) and as 'a "choice" borne out of constraint' (Graham, 2014). While it is also evident from the life story narratives in this book that all interviewees would have preferred to establish a family within a more traditional family setting, their narratives clearly illustrate that the meaning of real and ideal are transformed in the process towards motherhood. As shown in the exemplary narrative by Charlotte, the decision to embark upon solo motherhood is neither to be seen as plan A nor as a 'second best'. When the prospect of forming a nuclear family diminishes or ceases to exist, the change in circumstances makes biographical revisions necessary and a new ideal – in this case donor insemination – enters into the life planning process and into the process of negotiation and normalization as described above. Hence, the break between real and ideal are mended over time. The following passages are typical accounts in this regard:

> It's been my choice, but that's because my first choice failed somehow, at the time that it was relevant, and it's not because she is a second choice, that's not how it should be interpreted, but I would rather have been together with someone and had a real family, but that didn't happen, so now I'm going 200% all in on the family I have and defending it tooth and nail. But you know, it's been my choice, but I also haven't opted out of anything, because it's not like there were other options at the time.
> –Ditte (lawyer, daughter age 1 through ICSI)

> Of course having a child alone is not the first choice, that's not how it was. But having said that, in the process, it's like all of a sudden, the alternative stopped existing in my head, and I don't think of it as a second choice now, and I haven't for a long time, but of course, you know…I would have liked to have a man to have them with, but that didn't happen, and that's ok.
> –Cecilie (three-month old son through IVF)

> The more I'm in it, the more right it feels.
> –Anne (pharmaconomist, in treatment with IVF)

In a narrative account, one attempts to create a coherent and meaningful story using different narrative conventions and as such, to reconstruct and make sense of past experiences. Through the narration of turning points and biographical revisions, the women's biographical narratives detail main shifts in motivations, actions and choices, and while they include post-rationalizations of the ambivalence of choice because the interviewees have all moved past the process of decision-making and into the phase of treatment or the realization of motherhood, their narrative accounts reflect the meaning-making process they undergo from the point at which they begin contemplating the decision.

For Ditte, the ambivalence in choice is very much present in her narrative account, as seen above. The majority however, reflect retrospectively on the ambivalence of embarking upon solo motherhood and while ascribing different meaning to it, they all attach importance to the positive aspect of making what they believe to be the right choice. It is a choice made within certain circumstances but only one interviewee characterizes the decision as one made 'out of constraint'. For the remaining women, the choice is viewed and narratively presented as the best possible choice and one that is made through an act of agency rather than constraint. In general, the phase of contemplation, while sometimes lasting for years, does not form a strong presence in their narratives. For the women who have become mothers, the solo mother family constellation in particular is embraced wholeheartedly and 'defended tooth and nail', even though they still hope to find a partner eventually. This does not imply that all uncertainties disappear and that considerations about 'the need for a father' fade away, but they take on other guises, concerning managing the implications of the choice, as opposed to doubting the choice itself. They contemplate potential future questions from their children regarding the absence of the biological father for example, and consider how they will go about answering these types of questions in the best possible way.

The women's narration of the choice being neither their initial choice nor a second best could be termed a *'narrative of best choice'* to designate the duality characterizing the paradox of choice and the mitigation of tension between real and ideal. On the one hand, the choice is presented as a departure from the 'ideal' nuclear family construction and, with a view to individual wishes and societal concerns, their choice to contemplate solo motherhood is framed as being about the active choice to have a child and not the active choice not to have a partner. This distinction is quintessential to 'the narrative of best choice' because on the other hand, it is vital that the choice to contemplate solo motherhood is by design and not by chance and that the positive and active choice to pursue solo motherhood will form a part of the child's conception story. It is furthermore important that they are able to justify their choice and are committed to the decision. The 'best choice narrative' is a narrative about strategically managing preferred life plans according to accessible life chances and about minimizing the insecurities and ambivalences that not only follow from the edict to individually manage 'the reflexively organized trajectory of the self' (Giddens, 1991, p. 85) but that also follow from embarking upon a less 'standardized' route to family formation. Managing such insecurities leads back to the need to present and identify themselves (through both self and other identification) as being responsible and emotional mature women who are capable of handling the implications of this choice. Paradoxically, emphasizing the dualism of the choice being neither plan A nor 'second best', come to act as an adaptation strategy to integrate the changing conceptions of the ideal.

Several interviewees explicitly extend the ambivalence of choice to broader social trends and inscribe their own choice to embark upon solo motherhood within a greater single and individualized culture within which meeting a partner seem increasingly difficult. While they value the sociocultural and medical opportunities that have rendered possible their particular route to motherhood, they also express that it may be potentially worrisome for society in general if the trend of going it alone keep growing, because it for them reflects increasingly shared difficulties of meeting partners and forming families. Hence, while they point to individual motives and particular life trajectories, they also locate and position themselves within broader social trends and developments.

4.2.5 *Younger Solo Mothers*

In the interview study more than a third of the women are in their early thirties when they initiate treatment. Within a fertility treatment discourse, this is considered young because of the general tendency to be in your late thirties or older when treatment is initiated. At this point women are reported to find themselves at a stage where there is a strong feeling of 'last call' and 'time is running out' in terms of having a child of one's own. This tendency still seems to be endemic among single women pursuing solo motherhood through assisted conception. As the study by Salomon et al. showed, the 184 single women in the survey were – with an average age of 36.1 – 3.5 years older than the comparison group of cohabiting women. Still, if we look at the age distribution, 6% of the single women were below the age of 30, 19.6% were between the age of 30–34, 35.3% between the age of 35–37 and 39.1% between 38 and 40 (2015, p. 476). It is difficult however to document whether the group of single women have become younger over time in terms of commencing treatment. In the expert interview with Maria Salomon, she assesses that they see more younger women in treatment at the largest hospital in Denmark, Rigshospitalet (expert interview), and this is also a shared estimation among several of the interviewees in this study. Regardless of the potential increase, the question of why younger women embark upon solo motherhood remains salient. According to Salomon, younger single women also experience a feeling of time running out in terms of meeting the right partner and having time to have a child. Some for instance, have been diagnosed with PSO and know that it might be more difficult to conceive if they wait. Some women also want to have more than one child and know they cannot wait too long if they are to succeed (expert interview). These observations are also in keeping with the motivating factors expressed by the women in this study. In general, they do not seem to differ significantly from the common motivations mentioned above. Nonetheless, the wish to become a young mother and to potentially have more than one child are mentioned as main reasons to embark upon solo motherhood when the women are in their thirties. Interlinked with experiences of not having found the right partner and awareness of age-related infertility issues add to the shared feeling of being pressed for time.

As exemplified by Sarah's narrative, it generally seems to be slightly more difficult to legitimize the decision to embark upon solo motherhood at a younger age. Initiating treatment in one's early thirties or at a younger age – despite potential infertility issues, increasing concerns about fertility decline or the wish to have more than one child etc. – challenge to a greater extent, expectations inherent in the 'normal biography', and similarly to expectations underlying the age discourse within the fertility treatment system. Making the decision to embark upon solo motherhood in your early thirties signals a more active deselection of a partner as well as unexhausted options of finding one, than when the decision is made in your late thirties and seen as a 'last call' to have a child of your own. Based on a small observation study in a fertility clinic, expert and interviewee statements (see description of research, Appendix 1), these age-related expectations seem to be embedded in greater cultural expectations related to the structuring of 'normative life-events' (Heinz and Krüger, 2001, pp. 37–38). While they appear to be of more indirect character, they still pose a 'systemic contradiction' (Beck and Beck-Gernsheim, 2001). On the one hand, the 'age discourse' produces and reproduces a certain set of expectations as to the timing and sequencing of life transitions and on the other hand, there is a growing national trend of raising awareness about fertility reduction and associated risk factors as well as national campaigning encouraging citizens to start having children earlier in life. Increasing age constitutes a significant factor in terms of fertility decline, and the women in this study are generally very much aware of the risk of waiting. The 'biographical solution' to the contradiction (Beck and Beck-Gernsheim, 2001) implies for many of the younger women in this study, a redefinition of time pressure seen according to their own desires for a child and their current life situation. They stress the risks of waiting, substantiating this by drawing on the emerging narrative of fertility awareness and, as mentioned above, then rework the biographical order in terms of planning for a child first and potentially finding a partner afterwards.

4.3 Identifying as a Solo Mother – Terminology as Categorization

When the term 'single mothers by choice' was coined by Jane Mattes in 1982, the aim was to describe a group of responsible, mature and empowered women who *chose* to enter motherhood (Graham and Braverman, 2012). It furthermore served the aim of dissociating this group of women from the pejorative terminology historically associated with the term 'single mothers' (Bock, 2000). The terminology has caught on and alternative terms such as 'choice mother' and 'solo mother' are also applied. 'Solo mother' is the preferred term within the UK-based research, mainly in order to avoid the ambivalence associated with the 'by choice' connotation (Graham, 2013). In the Danish setting, both the terminology of solo mother and single mother by choice (in the Danish equivalent) are used. In keeping with the general literature within the field, I generally use the term solo mothers throughout the book as it appears to be a more neutral categorization. Still, while it is meant to situate the book within a particular field of research, draw attention to and provide knowledge about a 'phenomenon' less researched, it may paradoxically help to reproduce an understanding of 'solo mothers' as involving a single bounded group of women and to stress a fixed identity and fixed position within a certain type of family form. This is not the intention, and as previously defined (Chapter 2), I approach the concept of identity as a matter of identification that 'calls attention to complex (and often ambivalent) *processes*' (Brubaker and Cooper, 2000, p. 17). Hence, the aim is not to maintain solo motherhood as a 'fixed' and essentialized categorization and solo mothers as representing a 'unified subject'.

If we turn to the women in this book, the questions remains as to whether they identify according to the terminology of solo mothers or single mothers by choice? In general, they do not feel a strong need to dissociate themselves from being referred to as solo mothers or single mothers by choice, but most simply identify as mothers or mothers-to-be. In this regard, it is evident from the interviews that a strong 'groupist' sense of group-belonging (Brubaker and Cooper, 2000) does not form part of their self-understandings. In fact, the vast majority do not see themselves as being part of a distinct and confined group that share a specific set of attributes. Rather the concept of 'loosely affiliative' seems more adequate as they relate to the terminology and, as described above, many find it important to be able to broadly identify with others in similar family constellations or others in 'non-traditional' and/or 'new family' structures. Around a third of the women are in favour of the concept of solo mother/single mothers by choice to a point where they identify by it and use it to describe their own situation. The majority of women, however, do not use the terminology and are not comfortable being subjected to this specific classification. As Christina states,

> I think basically that [dissociating from other single mothers] is more about oneself - in terms of how you see others, because there are also single mothers that have separated from their husbands, who can be resourceful and there are also single women whose husbands have died, or who also are single mothers and are resourceful too, so I think, yeah, it's more about making it your own, and that you don't need to justify it to others via an expression, but that you are comfortable with the decision yourself, and that you can carry it, that's where the strength should come from. And then they can call me a single mother, or a solo mother, or they can think that I went out on the town and slept with a random guy, but if I know the background and am firm in my faith about it, then they can call me what they want, because it's just as legitimate as anything else, because it's about the choice I made, because I felt it was right.
> –Christina (social worker, in treatment with IVF)

Hence, the main imperative is being able to justify the decision to themselves and their children and as described above, self-identify as responsible and emotionally mature women. Within the main group of women who dissociate themselves from the solo mother label, a few explicitly state that it remains important to them to disseminate their situation as one that is 'by choice'. Identification is often about ambivalent processes as stated above, and while the majority do not feel the need to belong to the specific identity-category of solo mothers, they both adopt and challenge external processes of definition as described throughout this chapter. These are integrated in their self-understandings and into the decision-making process of justifying the choice as a moral and acceptable one. While they to a lesser extent locate abilities such as responsibility and emotional maturity, within the confines of the solo mother categorization – as reflected in the above passage from Christina - they both implicitly and explicitly draw on moral distinctions in positioning themselves as qualified parents and in identifying a number of personal abilities and criteria for good mothering. Some explicitly question the absence of a 'screening process' by one's general practitioner prior to fertility treatment and call for a greater debate about the issue of parenting capacity.[2] Here, the main point raised is that parenting in general, and solo parenthood in particular, requires a certain set of resources and skills to meet the needs of a child.

4.4 Claiming Family in Terms of Acceptance, Rights and Benefits

The availability of rights and benefits are important aspects of being able to 'claim family' and likewise imperative to the experience of one's particular family constellation being culturally accepted and recognized (May, 2015, p. 483). The 2007 legislative change in which single and lesbian women in Denmark gained the legislative right to assisted reproduction manifests as one of the most decisive developments at the societal level when contemplating solo motherhood. The attainment of equal rights within the area, and consequently the possibility of undergoing treatment in public clinics signifies a cultural acceptance of lesbian and solo mother families. It supports the women's individual view that solo motherhood is a viable, moral and acceptable route to motherhood and to the increasing legitimization and normalization of this particular family constellation. The legislative, medical and financial options provided within the framework of the Danish welfare state are addressed by the interviewees as privileges and resources that support the realization of the solo mother family.

The financial support available in terms of public fertility treatment and additional child benefits are highly appreciated but they have not been decisive in the decision-making process. To the contrary, the women in this study have been prepared to pay for treatment themselves, as some have done, and the decision to contemplate solo motherhood has been incumbent on securing a permanent job and being self-supporting as described above. From January 2014, solo mothers who have conceived through donor insemination were granted a 'special grant' for single providers. The women appreciate the extra child benefits provided but do not take them for granted or regard them as pre-requisites; rather they are seen as extra resources to support their children or children-to-be.

Prior to 2014, this particular grant was only offered to single providers if one or both parents to the child in question were deceased, or if the father was unknown. The difference in benefits provoked debate, and several interviewees explicitly refer to its discriminatory effects; not in terms of the financial aspect but in terms of its symbolic meaning. It was perceived as non-recognition of donor-conceived children compared to children with unknown fathers due to other circumstances, thus implicitly and normatively rendering the donor insemination route to single motherhood less legitimate and accepted.

---

[2]The law on assisted reproduction requires that the attending doctor and not the GP assess parental fitness.

The *equality* in terms of rights and benefits is, in both its de jure and de facto designations, the most important social change mentioned when the interviewed women are asked whether any societal developments and conditions have influenced their decision to contemplate solo motherhood. Other resources such as public fertility treatment, public day care options, child benefits, access to leave schemes etc. do not enter into the decision-making process because the women emphasize the need to be self-supporting and because, when asked about it, they focus on resources and changes that are particular to forming solo mother families and which do not include more general welfare state resources. For instance, public care options are broadly available and the majority of parents rely on them, as mentioned by some. Still, the choice to embark upon solo motherhood is less 'stratified' in a Danish sociocultural context compared to the UK for instance, due to the level of public support provided. In the UK, as mentioned previously, the choice to embark upon solo motherhood comes across as more ambivalent and seems to be less culturally accepted than in Denmark. One could argue that the difference in 'stratification' and public support constitutes one sociocultural explanation of the difference in terms of the ambivalence of choice and in the level of cultural acceptance (Graham and Ravn, 2016).

4.5 Relating the Personal and Social: A Model of the Decision-Making Process

The decision to embark upon solo motherhood is shaped by a number of complex motivations, biographical particulars/commonalities and sociocultural narratives that collectively and interrelatedly influence the decision-making process. In this process, past experiences and turning points related to relationship story, fertility issues and future anticipations of family life, among others, provide grounds for present motivations, rationales and strategies that include biographical revisions and a reworking of biographical elements in terms of prioritizing having a child of one's own before finding a partner. This shared plot twist serves as a strategy to mend 'biographical discontinuity' (Tjørnhøj-Thomsen, 2003, p. 64) and to minimize the tension between conceptions of ideals and of present realities.

The model below (Fig. 4.1) provides an overview of the many factors that enter into the decision-making process. In the interlinking of past experiences, current motivations and future anticipations of family formation, the position of motherhood remains a strong identifier throughout the biographical narratives and appears impossible to transcend. It is projected into future visions of motherhood, and current self-understandings and life plans are transformed accordingly (see centreline, turning points → motivations → effects). This identification can be argued to be compounded by the fact that when embarking upon fertility treatment, potential parents are expected to be deeply committed to parenting, creating what Faircloth and Gürtin has termed 'pre-conception' parents (in Graham, 2018, p. 252). Hence, both individual, societal and technological expectations of motherhood consolidate the strong identification of becoming a mother in the future.

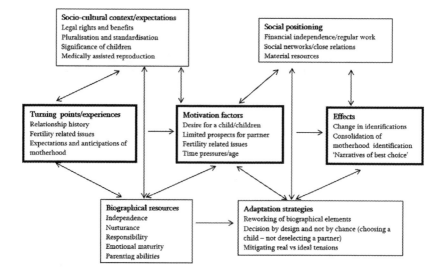

Fig. 4.1.   The Decision-Making Process: Relating the Personal
and the Social.

In a simplified way, the model furthermore illustrates the main interlinkages between biographical resources/social positionings and sociocultural conditions/ main narratives. For instance, the attainment of equal rights and benefits have added to the women's notions of solo motherhood being a viable, moral and acceptable route to motherhood and to the increasing legitimization and normalization of this particular family constellation (as reflected by legislation and expressed in the expert/biographical interviews). The increasing normalization of 'non-traditional families' such as the blended family model is seen as having expanded the possibilities for adopting new subject positions and for 'doing family' in new ways, and these developments broadly act as a way to rationalize their choice. At the same time, to legitimize and normalize the choice of forming solo mother families, the women also continuously enter into dialogue with more estab-lished and accepted cultural models for family and kinship formation, navigating between concurrent biographical trends of pluralization and standardization.

Chapter 5

Undergoing Fertility Treatment: Reworking Boundaries of 'Natural Processes'

While medically assisted reproduction has both a destabilizing and generative impact on cultural settings, social relations and our cultural construction of self, it is also itself shaped by economic, cultural, political and moral surroundings, as well as the recipients who appropriate these technologies into their lives (Becker, 2000; Inhorn and Birenbaum-Carmeli, 2008; Markussen and Gad, 2007; Thompson, 2005). On the one hand, then, innovations within the field of reproductive technologies have helped redefine and stretch the limits of our normative understandings of natural facts and given rise to new understandings of, for instance, procreation and family formations (Franklin, 1993, 2013b; Inhorn and Birenbaum-Carmeli, 2008). On the other hand, they have also been foundational in securing clear legal demarcations between the 'natural' and the 'artificial' (see Chapter 3) and in safe-guarding 'naturalized' ideas about biological processes and kinship relations.

The following Chapter 6 on 'forming donor-conceived families' will examine how these tensions affect normalization and naturalization processes in terms of how biological and social aspects of kinship are both sustained and re-defined in complex ways as biographical revisions take place. In Chapter 6, I argue that the issue of transgressing boundaries in the process towards motherhood closely interlinks with the process of undergoing fertility treatment. In this chapter, I expand on this argument and explore how the interviewed women perceive and engage with medically assisted reproduction, and in what way processes of fertility treatment influence their life planning and biographical revisions. I also turn to both the physical and emotional experiences of undergoing treatment and discuss both material and discursive processes in terms of fertility treatment. I ask for instance, whether the women in this study change their perception of reproductive technology during their process of treatment and how they cope with undergoing treatment without a partner. Furthermore, I ask in what way the above-mentioned processes of naturalization and normalization intertwine with 'technology as culture' (Becker, 2000, p. 237) as depending on the meanings assigned to reproductive technologies.

5.1 Treatment Procedures, Risks and Success Rates

Today, the field of medically assisted reproduction (MAR), and the technolog-ization of human reproduction is a phenomenon which is both 'ordinary and

Lived Realities of Solo Motherhood, Donor Conception
and Medically Assisted Reproduction, 105–125
Copyright © 2021 Tine Ravn
Published under exclusive licence by Emerald Publishing Limited
doi:10.1108/978-1-83909-115-520211007

curious' (Franklin, 2013a). Curious because it remains paradoxical, and ordinary, because having a child via the aid of assisted reproduction has become increasingly normalized (as previously noted, in Denmark, 10.5% of babies born yearly (2019 estimate) come into the world as a result of assisted reproduction (Danish Fertility Society, 2020a). As described in the introduction to this book, MAR includes all ART procedures as well as intra-uterine insemination with partner or donor sperm (IUI-H, IUI-D). ART procedures cover 'all interventions that include the in-vitro handling of both human oocytes and sperm or embryos for the purpose of reproduction'. These may include IVF, embryo transfer ET, intra-cytoplasmic sperm injection ICSI and gamete and embryo cryopreservation (Zegers-Hochschild et al., 2017, p. 1790). Despite substantial regional variation in practices and outcomes, the use of ART has increased and worldwide, it is estimated that 2.4 million ART cycles are carried out each year resulting in approximately 500,000 babies born. Spain, followed by France, Germany, Italy and the UK are the most active IVF countries in Europe. ICSI is a procedure at where a single sperm cell is microinjected directly into the egg. ICSI was developed to counter male-factor infertility, for instance in the case of low sperm count. ICSI is a more costly and invasive procedure than conventional IVF, but applied with the rationale to produce higher fertilization rates, also in cases with no male infertility factors. Today, ICSI comprises the most common fertilization technique worldwide and is applied in the majority of IVF cases (Kushnir et al., 2017; ESHRE, 2020; Wang and Sauer, 2006; Zegers-Hochschild et al., 2017; Dang et al., 2019).

Half of the women in this research have applied donor insemination (IUI-D) at the time of interview and the other half have undergone IVF treatment (ICSI has been applied in three cases, see overview in Appendix 1). In Denmark, insemination is first-line treatment. If this treatment is unsuccessful or is known not to have an effect due to various conditions, IVF treatment with or without ICSI is accessible. Up to six rounds of insemination and up to three rounds of IVF can be offered in the public health care system. Treatment are offered for the woman's first child (frozen embryo replacement (FER) can be offered for a second child) and for women below the age of 41 (46 in private fertility clinics). Fertility treatment in the public health care sector is free of charge. The costs for fertility medicine are not covered but subsidies can be applied for (The Danish Health Data Authority, 2020; Ernst, 2020).

5.1.1 Success Rates and Risks of Treatment

For people undergoing treatment, advancements and improvement in techniques and clinical procedures, have increased the success rates of treatment and chances of a live birth, despite great variation worldwide. Data from the British Human Fertilisation & Embryology Authority (HFEA) shows that this is the case for all patients below 43 years of age. IVF birth rates for women below the age of 35 were 31% per embryo transferred in 2018. For women aged 43 and above, the birth rates have remained below 5% per embryo transferred when the women in treatment use their own eggs. On average, the use of donor eggs can increase the success rate to above 20% for this group of women. In 2018, 18% of the women above the age of 40 used donor eggs (HFEA, 2020a; Chambers et al., 2016). In 2018, data from the Danish Health Data Authority shows that around a fourth of all IVF/ICSI treatments results in a clinical pregnancy for women below the age of 35. Age is an important factor for the success of treatment. Hence, for women between the age of 35 and 40, the success rate decreases to 17.9% and to 9.2% for women above the age of 40. For donor insemination, the success rate is 11.2% for women below the age of 40 and 5.3% for women above (The Danish Health Data Authority, 2020). In comparison, 2016 world data reported from ESHRE establishes the delivery rate from ART treatment to be 21.8% per aspiration and 28.9 cumulative.[1] For the long-term chances of having a child via fertility treatment, a Danish register-based national cohort study has found that the changes to conceive a child within a five-year period is 64% for women below 35 years, 49% for women between the age of 35 and 39, and 16% for women above the age of 40 (Malchau et al., 2017).

Overall, fertility treatment is considered safe and the procedures well tested. However, a number of risks are associated with treatment. The greatest complication of IVF is considered to be ovarian hyper stimulation (OHSS) at where too many eggs develop in the ovaries. Symptoms, among others, include abdominal discomfort, bloating and nausea. Severe cases are rare but potentially dangerous. Other associated risks are a slightly higher risk of an ectopic pregnancy (i.e. a pregnancy occurring in the fallopian tubes rather than in the womb) and pelvic inflammatory disease. After IVF treatment, the most significant risk is having a multiple pregnancy and birth as it increases the risks of miscarriage and premature births, among other complications. Despite cross-country variation in the number of embryos transferred, guidelines and calls for single-embryo transfer (SET) have resulted in a decrease in multiple births. Women who are above the age of 35 are at greater risk of complications such as miscarriages and pre-term birth. Birth defects are rare and it is not yet established whether they are caused by the treatment process or by infertility issues (HFEA, 2020b; Baldwin, 2019; NHS, 2020; ESHRE, 2020; Rigshospitalet, 2017; Klitzman, 2016). An increasing number of Danish and international studies have researched the psychosocial consequences of experiencing infertility and undergoing fertility treatment for couples and it is by now well-established that there is an increased risk of stress, anxiety and symptoms of depression associated with these circumstances. Contrary to other European countries such as Sweden, Belgium, Germany and the UK, which offer emotional patient counselling, mental health professionals that attend to the psychosocial consequences of infertility and fertility treatment, do not form part of the healthcare personal at Danish fertility clinics (Schmidt and Sejbæk, 2012).

---

[1] 'The number of deliveries with at least one live birth resulting from one initiated or aspirated ART cycle, including all cycles in which fresh and/or frozen embryos are transferred, until one delivery with a live birth occurs or until all embryos are used, whichever occurs first' (Zegers-Hochschild et al., 2017, p. 1792).

5.2 Narratives on Undergoing Fertility Treatment

Below, three short and exemplary narratives foregrounding experiences of undergoing fertility treatment are included. They are exemplary in the sense that they detail central cross-sample themes of importance to explore the argument and objectives stated above. In addition, they explore the lived realities of assisted reproduction from different perspectives and phases related to treatment and treatment termination. Following the tripartite division of interviewees according to whether they are in fertility treatment, are pregnant or have become mothers through both IUI and/or IVF/ICSI, the three short and predominantly descriptive narratives offer perspectives from each of the three dimensions. The aim is to demonstrate both individual and the shared processual elements of undergoing treatment, and to explore how treatment experiences unfold and are emphasized both prospectively and retrospectively depending on whether treatment has been just initiated or has resulted in the realization of motherhood, for instance. In addressing some of the main themes to be further examined throughout this chapter, the narratives interweave personal and biographical features with matters of biology, discursive practices and reproductive technology.

5.2.1 In Fertility Treatment with IVF: Anne

Anne, 39, works as a pharmaconomist in a biotech company and lives north of Copenhagen. At the age of 34, she divorced her husband, and after a period of unsuccessful dating, she began to contemplate solo motherhood. At the age of 37, she discovered that she would need to undergo IVF treatment in order to become pregnant due to her having blocked fallopian tubes. For Anne, this acts as a catalytic event to starting treatment. At the time of the interview, she is a year into treatment and at this point in time she has completed five rounds of unsuccessful IVF treatments.

   Treatment round number three did not result in a fertilized egg and she is offered another round of treatment, however the medical staff recommend that she have her fallopian tubes removed to increase the chance of success. After her operation, she undergoes another round of IVF and this results in an unsuccessful biochemical pregnancy. It is standard procedure to be offered three rounds of IVF treatment in the public system (cf. above) but due to her evidently now being able to become pregnant, Anne is offered one last round of treatment. It does not result in a pregnancy, and her course of treatment in the public medical system is terminated. In narrating her experience of going through IVF treatment, including undergoing hormone stimulation, Anne states:

> So yeah, the hormones are really bad, it's unbelievably difficult. I feel like I can't control who I am at all, because I just get in such bad moods. Of course, I also think that's where the psychological element comes in, that you're just waiting, and then you have to go in for scan and then wait, and then go for another scan, and it's all so, it's all so laborious. It's ridiculous to have eggs taken out, well

it takes up a whole day and it's bloody painful, and that same time you feel guilty about all the time you're not at work, and it's really… you really really really need to want it for it to be worth it. And then I think about the fact that it's harder because I'm doing it alone, well I don't know what it would be like if I was doing it with a partner, then you'd have someone to share it with. […] The worst thing about the hormones is that you know, every time you try, it gets worse, because they give you more and more. […] So, but it's just…that's how it is, I don't have any other options. So that's, that's just how it is. Yeah.

When speaking about her process of going through treatment, Anne also tells of gradually becoming more familiar with the medical treatment procedures and practices at the fertility clinic. Prior to initiating treatment, Anne narrates that she believed it to be a matter of simply becoming pregnant after a short period of time:

So, I chose the donor I wanted, then I just had to have all that IVF, and then I would become pregnant. And I had absolutely no idea what I was getting myself into. And I had to, well the whole thing about having to inject myself, I totally hated it, it was just the worst nightmare, and I felt so ill.

Later in the interview, she retrospectively recounts:

Because the further into the process you get, the more you kind of, well you get so desperate, because you think to yourself, I just need to have this baby, I don't care how, I just need to have this baby. So the last two times I've been into the hospital, I've just said 'I want a donor that can make babies', and they were like, 'we can't just say that'. Then I said 'now listen, I know how it works in here' – you get smarter, the further into the process you get, you know?

Anne has decided to continue IVF treatment in a private clinic. She has money saved up and is not prepared to 'give up' on having a child of her own. She has also considered the option of double donation but she has not yet decided on how long she will continue in her quest for a child.

5.2.2 *Pregnant through IUI-D: Marie Louise*

Marie Louise, 29, lives in Aarhus and is a lecturer in child psychology/pedagogy (see also her biographical narrative in Chapter 6). At the time of the interview, she is six weeks pregnant after her first round of treatment with donor insemination (IUI-D). After receiving her referral for fertility treatment, Marie Louise embarks upon treatment at a private clinic because she wishes to use an open donor. After her initial appointment, she finds out that the donor legislation has been changed and is referred to treatment in a public fertility clinic. Before insemination she is tested through the procedure of hysterosalpingography (HSG) in order to see if there is clear passage through at least one of her fallopian tubes. When describing going through this test, Marie Louise states:

> It was great to see the light of the substance in my ovaries, that I could see that it was just as it should be, and that it folded out on the screen in front of me, proud and happy, thinking this is going to happen, because I'm super-fertile!

As part of the donor insemination procedure, an initial ultra sound scan takes place in order to monitor the amount and size of follicles present. At the first ultrasound of her ovaries, Marie Louise tells that 'the doctor found one amazingly great egg at 1.8 mm in diameter'. Following an ovulation injection that secures that ovulation has taken place, Marie Louise is inseminated with donor semen. At this session, she discusses the next step in her treatment procedure with the doctor, should the first round of insemination be unsuccessful. The doctor suggests that Marie Louise begins hormone stimulation after a second round of insemination. As a response to this suggestion, Marie Louise narrates the following:

> So I said to her, 'Well I don't want that, I don't want hormones'. Then she said that we have to make a long-term plan for you, and we strongly recommend that you take hormones, so I said no, I'm young, I'm not 40 and I don't want hormones, it's unnatural and I want to do it on my own. I don't want an increased risk of having triplets. And I'm quite sure my body will help me, so I'm not there right now, so then she said 'No, but you probably will be after your second attempt, if it hasn't worked', and I said I thought that was a bit much […].

Marie Louise agrees to the plan but narrates:

> I wouldn't say it to her but deep down, I'd always felt like this, my idea was that I would give it a try without hormones, and if it didn't work, then I'd have to wait and see if I met a man and if it worked with him. Because I didn't want to get involved in hormones and in vitro fertilization and be made infertile because I was quite sure that that wasn't what it was based on. So I wasn't ready.

Later in the interview she tells:

> I've always had a feeling that I could do this. And in any case, I wanted to be able to have some proper attempts even with the

poor odds, I still wanted to have at least three tries without them pouring hormones and other things into me, but I also have to say that I can see that the desire to actually get pregnant increased in the process – that you're so close and you're in the middle of it all. So maybe I would have changed my mind about taking hormones anyway, but I just think, when you know how hard it is to take hormones and how much it affects you psychologically, and that I'm alone – I don't have anyone to get annoyed or angry at, or to cry on or laugh with in my private everyday life [...] Because I know full well that I have an ovulation injection and insemination instruments involved in the process, but I just wanted to do it in a normal way. That meant something to me.

Subsequently she states:

Yeah, I think also that I say that it happened normally, but it wasn't in any way natural, it was totally technological. I'm so happy about that. I love technology, and I just don't know where the boundary should be.

5.2.3 Mother to a Child Conceived through IVF: Cecilie

Cecilie, 36, lives in Copenhagen where she works as a nurse. At the age of 34, she initiates fertility treatment after two consecutive relationships have ended. Cecilie cannot imagine herself not becoming a mother and she does not want to wait too long due to considerations about fertility decline. In this regard she also states that she does not want to be pressed for time in case she needs to pursue other options or wants to have more than one child. Cecilie undergoes six rounds of insemination and due to a condition of PCO, is also treated with hormone stimulation. The insemination procedures do not result in a pregnancy, and Cecilie continues with IVF treatment. In terms of moving on from insemination to IVF treatment, Cecilie asserts:

Well I don't really think I thought it would work with insemination, then we just had to get on with the next option, and for me, it's not like it was a bad experience, it was fine. Well, you're a bit worried the first time you have to have eggs taken out, it's like, how's it going to feel? And then the next thing, are any of them going to get fertilised? So there are lots of phases, where there are these concerns which are unclear, but I also think it gave renewed hope to get started with it, because all else being equal, the chance of getting pregnant is greater, so that probably gave me a little new hope, I probably didn't believe in it before, no ...

In recapitulating the process of undergoing IVF, she narrates:

> So we started IVF, with hormone treatment and everything, and then it was in, was it in August? It was August or the beginning of September '13 that I had the first eggs taken out, and I can't remember if it was seven or nine eggs, one of the two anyway, and then you're on tenterhooks while you wait to find out if any of them have been fertilized, and there were three of them that had been, but then they were two-celled. They hadn't divided that much, so they recommended that I should have them inserted anyway, so I did, and then I was, well, I didn't get pregnant from them. And then there was one egg left that had been frozen and I had that inserted mid-November and then there was luck. Yeah, it was unbelievable that there was just one little frozen egg left, and I didn't believe in it at all, I was a bit annoyed that we couldn't just move on to the next option because if two fresh ones couldn't make it up there, it would be weird if this one could! So I was half annoyed, but I've never been so happy to be wrong! *Laughs* Yeah, so that was a bit crazy, so I had it, I think it was mid-November I had it inserted and then I found out 14 days later that I was pregnant, yeah.

When asked about her experiences of undergoing hormone treatment, Cecilie gives the following account:

> You get kind of half-crazy being in this fertility process, you know? Because it's just difficult, you know? Because being in the process, I'd been in the process for a while by then, and I just wanted it so much, so I think it was more these things, and they still affect me a bit when I think about it, kind of mood-related, that I probably... But it wasn't like it was completely unbearable, no, it wasn't. [...] What I remember most clearly, it wasn't so much the reaction, it was more the ups and downs and the hope, and the 'It didn't happen...' That was hard, and then there was the anxiety about if it's going to work. If only you could know that it would happen, then you could handle it taking time, but that I found really hard because I didn't dare, no I didn't dare to think, what if I can't? I couldn't really face that that was a possibility. And luckily it didn't happen!

5.2.4 The Process of Fertility Treatment: Narrative Cross-cutting Themes

The three short and descriptive biographical narratives include a number of key themes that emerge across the complete set of individual narratives:

5.2.4.1 Physical and Emotional Strain of Undergoing Fertility Treatment
All three narratives include the joint physical and emotional strain of undergoing fertility treatment and its interlinkage to doing it alone without a partner with whom to share the experience. Cecilie and Anne experience the bodily strain of hormone treatment in various ways but both focus on the emotional 'ups and downs' that characterize the process. As to the latter, many explicitly describe the process as a 'roller-coaster' ride in constantly vacillating between hope and discouragement.

5.2.4.2 Processual 'Roller-coaster' Effects
In this regard several women tell of being reluctant to plan treatment ahead out of fear that the current round of treatment will not be successful. In Cecilie's case, she experienced renewed hope of achieving a pregnancy when she moved on from insemination to IVF, and Anne tells of becoming more desperate for a child as she progresses through unsuccessful rounds of treatments. Marie Louise becomes pregnant in her very first insemination attempt but narrates how she experienced an increased desire for a child during this process.

5.2.4.3 The 'Open-endedness' of Treatment
This speaks to the issue of redefining one's boundaries for accepted treatment procedures when moving through the process. The desire for a child rarely decreases and the options of untested procedures, new statistics and success rates add to a 'culture of perseverance' as Thompson denotes the 'open-ended' nature of treatment in which new options open up if one's age and financial situation allows it (2005, pp. 94–95). This processual open-endedness also characterizes many of the narratives in this study and in particular from the women who are or have gone through several rounds of treatment.

5.2.4.4 Enacting Agency
This also relates to the process of 'getting smarter' during the process, as Anne states when referring to the process of gradually becoming more thoroughly versed in the established procedures, practices and possibilities of the medical system. It adds to the theme of exercising agency when navigating within the medical treatment system and through the various processes of treatment, and relates to the ontological transformations that takes place during treatment (Thompson, 2005).

The main themes identified and delineated above will be expanded upon in the following sections.

5.3 Navigating the 'Roller Coaster' Process of Fertility Treatment

The process of undergoing fertility treatment, and in particular IVF treatment, has been described as an 'emotional roller-coaster' (Thompson, 2005, p. 93); as becoming a 'way of life' (Franklin, 1997, p. 131) and reproductive technology as a 'catalyst for disruption' (Becker, 2000, p. 266) in terms of its emotional and physical impacts. In a review of 25 years' research into 'women's emotional adjustment to IVF', it is found that negative emotions increase concurrently with unsuccessful treatment cycles and that these emotions are highly linked to the threat of treatment failure (Verhaak et al., 2007). The roller-coaster metaphor is explicitly invoked by several of the women in this research to describe the stress and strain related to continuously experiencing alternating states of hope and discouragement in the treatment process which – as also demonstrated above – is strongly interlinked with the unendurable thought that treatment may not result in pregnancy and a child of one's own.

Three decades ago, Sarah Franklin described IVF technology as a 'hope technology', (1997, p. 192; 2013a) and despite – or because of – new and improved techniques, enhanced success rates and new visions of progress, reproductive technologies continue to epitomize the hope of a successful outcome. Hope in this regard is not to be confused with naive expectations regarding treatment outcomes or an expression of an incessant state of emotion. Reproductive technologies are also always imbued with ambivalence and con-tradictory states of emotion (Franklin, 2013a, pp. 7–8). In this study, we see this duality most clearly expressed through the use of the 'roller-coaster' metaphor or the similar expression of processual 'ups and downs'.

In the narrative interviews the 'roller-coaster' metaphor is used as a more general characteristic of the treatment process, and I was surprised to observe it manifest so intensively within a single treatment procedure. When I visited the Fertility Clinic at Aarhus University Hospital, I was present during an egg-retrieval surgery. During an egg-retrieval procedure, the woman is awake but is given various pain-relieving medications. By means of ultrasound guidance, a needle is passed to the ovaries and follicles, and the latter are aspirated and sucked into a test tube. Following this, a biomedical laboratory technician examines the fluid microscopically to identify the egg. Not all follicles contain a mature egg and if this is the case, it will be categorized as 'empty'. In general 10–12 eggs will be retrieved but the number can vary from a couple of eggs to 20–30 in total.

The egg retrieval procedure, I experienced was with a couple in their thirties. I was later told that they had been through a trying process in order to become parents, and I remember clearly noticing the tension present when I entered the surgery room together with the physician who was going to perform the surgical procedure. At the beginning of the egg-retrieval, no eggs could be identified and the situation grew more and more intense. It was a very emotionally charged situation, not only for the couple but for everyone present in the room, and it was with bated breath that everyone waited for the laboratory technician to give a status on the fluid examinations. After a while, the technician enthusiastically yelled 'there is an egg' and the atmosphere changed a little and became briefly more optimistic, but the oscillation between an atmosphere of despair and hope continued, and the intensity of it was overwhelming. In this specific case the 'emotional roller-coaster' (Thompson, 2005, p. 93) may represent a microcosm of the greater IVF treatment process or may merely characterize the single procedure. Taking into account the couple's medical history, the former seems to be a reasonable assumption. However, the point I wish to make here is that the alternating states of hope of despair played out even within minutes make great demands on patient's emotional endurance.

While the women in this study experience the emotional toll of treatment in various ways – experiences that also depend on their different biographical stories, their medical situation (e.g. regarding whether or not they have been diagnosed with infertility issues) and the bodily reactions to treatment – I generally find that while the physical and emotional strain reinforce each other (see below), it is the emotional stress of 'not knowing' that causes the greatest strain and vulnerability. The stakes are very high because IVF is seen as more or less the last option in order to have an own child. There is also the possibility of embarking upon double donation, but as discussed in the following chapter, this option triggers a new set of ethical considerations related to the social and bio-genetic aspects of kinship and family formation.

In her UK based study on solo motherhood, Graham finds that the ambivalence experienced in the decision-making process cease when the participants in her repeat-interview study enter into treatment (2013, see also previous references). Similarly, I also find that the insecurities experienced regarding the choice to pursue this route to motherhood transforms into an insecurity about the success of the treatment procedures. Graham also demonstrates how ethical concerns regarding the choice to embark upon solo motherhood are revisited in breaks between treatment and some of the initial moral concerns are 're-triggered' (2013, p. 137). In contrast, I do not generally see a similar process of re-rationalizing the choice once treatment is initiated. Rather, at this point in the process, the women in this research appear to be confident and comfortable with their choice, and supported by the 'open ended' nature of fertility treatment (Thompson, 2005, p. 94), it is the wish for a child that 'takes over' (Franklin, 1997, p. 131). The phase from decision-making to treatment can be regarded as a kind of 'liminal space' or 'between space' (Cobb in Laws and Rein, 2003, p. 205), in which the women's biographical revisions related to fully embarking upon solo motherhood have not yet, and may not be, realized. In this regard, Christina narrates the following:

> It's psychologically difficult to be in these situations with hormone treatment, and being in a waiting position, it worked – it didn't work, like all the time. At any rate, this is distressing.
> –Christina (Social worker, in treatment with IVF)

5.3.1 Undergoing Treatment as a Single Woman

When considering the observation above regarding the couple in treatment and the prefatory statements about undergoing treatment alone, a comparison between the emotional strains of treatment could be relevant. However, the single-case research design of this research does not allow for an assessment between undergoing treatment alone compared to experiencing treatment with a partner. At the same time, as this, to my understanding, is the first study to provide a detailed examination of how single women experience MAR treatment, it adds to the research on psychosocial consequences of infertility and treatment, showing that MAR treatment is also a severe stressor for single women undergoing treatment.

Some of the women imagine it to be harder to go it alone due to the lack of emotional support from a partner when greater decisions have to be made, for instance. Such decisions could be the number of embryos to be transferred (e.g. concerns about success rate and multiple births) or the decision on how long to continue treatment. The latter decision was also assessed by a nurse at the Fertility Clinic at Aarhus University Hospital to be more difficult to manage as a single woman undergoing treatment. In general, however, the aspect of going through treatment alone does not take up much space in their narratives on undergoing treatment. Possibly because the decision to do it alone has been comfortably made at this stage in the process as described above, and appears to be addressed as a matter-of-fact to which they plan accordingly. For instance, many tell of bringing close friends, mothers, sisters, or other close relations with them to the different treatment procedures for emotional support. Several also tell that this need is more discernible in the beginning of the treatment process, when the various procedures and practices are still new and unfamiliar.

5.3.2 A 'Rollercoaster' and a 'Conveyer-belt Life': Paradoxical Features of Treatment

As to the process of gradually becoming more familiar with the various fertility treatment procedures and practices, Ditte describes the following:

> I have to admit that I still remember that pretty clearly, picking up the phone the first time to call [the clinic], that was a massive struggle to overcome for me, because it was like, 'Now I'm taking the first step' and I have no idea what I'm getting myself involved in! […], and I remember when I went in the first time, I can almost remember how many steps there were on the way up, because it was like, shit man! And then you leave and you think, 'I'm pregnant, I'm pregnant!' And you're not at all, because it doesn't work, but it took a giant giant struggle for me, and from there it was much easier, because then I was, then I was in it – then the machine was in motion!
>
> –Ditte (Lawyer, daughter age 1 through ICSI)

First, setting the 'machine in motion' refers to the potentially overwhelming transition from decision to treatment. Second it refers to the greater machinery of the medical system and hence to the many working procedures and the general institutionalized and established-ways-of-doing-things (Jenkins, 2008, p. 40) within the particular field of fertility treatment. Many of the women who have undergone IVF treatment explicitly use descriptive words such as 'machine' and 'mechanical' to characterize the system and their individual treatment trajectory. The latter is foundational to the third and interrelated meaning of 'machine in motion'. Initiating fertility treatment implies enrolling oneself into a planned process of laborious and careful timetables that coordinate a number of activities and procedures. IUI treatments for instance include ultrasound scans, hormone stimulations (if fertility issues exist or if the first approximately three rounds of treatments in natural cycles do not result in a pregnancy), ovarian stimulation injection, insemination and pregnancy test. During IVF treatments, these procedures include initial examinations, hormone injections (short or long protocol), ultrasound scans, ovarian stimulation injections, egg retrieval/embryo transfer, pregnancy tests etc. As Thilde describes below, fertility treatment implies living in intervals:

> I'm a nurse and I want to understand a lot, but I think I disconnected a little at the end. At the end, I more or less followed the recommendations, because I couldn't really cope with any more, I couldn't, well I knew so much and had read so much, but I couldn't do it any more, because emotions play a huge part in it. And I also had some, well, some breaks in between when I wasn't in treatment, where I was, well there was a total relief not to live in 14 day intervals, you know? Because you live, you get your period, you start to take the medication, then you get to ovulation, then to the end of ovulation, then you either have some taken out or put in, and then you wait 14 days again, and those 14…ahhhh, and then you get your period, and then 14 days again, and 14, well you end up going crazy living like that. This fertility treatment is only for strong women, like I normally say.
>
> –Thilde (Nurse, 3 month-old son through IVF/ICSI)

Thilde's statement about disconnecting herself from the end of the process refers to the emotional strain of undergoing treatment (see below) but also speaks to the general issue of becoming more instrumental in one's approach during the course of treatment. The 'mechanical' and 'clinical' character of the process, experiences of unsuccessful cycles, change of donors, constant periods of waiting, and the increasing concerns about treatment failure, are aspects that add to this instrumentalization and increasing focus on the end goal of treatment. It also comes across as a coping mechanism to endure the emotional strain of treatment and stress related to the 'emotional roller-coaster' that comprises the physical and emotional reactions as well as the practical aspects of managing treatment logistics (Thompson, 2005, p. 93).

> It's a roller coaster ride all the way, and a train travelling ridiculously fast, that you can't get on, so it just drives on past… and at the same time it's also mechanical, it's such a difficult psychological process, and at the same time it's so mechanical in

the way you have to do this, and then you have to do this, and
there's no one that asks, 'how are you doing in all of this?' No, you
have to say that yourself.
                    –Christina (Social worker, in treatment with IVF)

Christina describes the paradoxical feature of fertility treatment being both
'mechanical' and linear in nature while at the same time causing a number of
emotional and bodily non-linear 'ups and downs'. As Charlotte describes below, such
emotional disruptions may also occur from the outset of the treatment procedure:

I'm not willing to go through anything, but I'm ready to try a lot
to get pregnant, and I think well, fantastic that there's this
possibility, imagine if there wasn't. So of course it also plays a
part, that there's this huge process and I'm thinking I'm not so far
into it yet that I can tell how it is, but I've had one attempt and
even without hormones, it's quite a rollercoaster ride mentally –
vulnerable and all those kinds of things – so then I wonder, whoah,
what would it be like if you're affected by hormones?
                    –Charlotte (Physiotherapist, in treatment with IUI-D)

To understand better how emotional and physical processes interlink and
compound each other, a comparison of women undergoing IVF treatment for the
purpose of either becoming pregnant or donating eggs proves illustrative. Cooper
and Waldby (2014) compare Almeling's study on egg vending (2011) with studies
of patients undergoing fertility treatment to become pregnant. They find that
'being paid to provide oocytes is a qualitatively different experience from that of
women using the same technology to try for pregnancy' (Cooper and Waldby,
2014, p. 51). Whereas egg donors referred to the treatment process in an
uncomplicated way with minimum reference to emotional strain or bodily
discomfort, fertility patients, on the other hand, stressed the emotional hardship,
the 'roller-coaster' process and the unpleasant physical effects (Cooper and
Waldby, 2014, pp. 51–53). In a recent survey by Almeling and Willey, the 'bodily
experiences of IVF' for the two groups is compared and they also finds that egg
donors' experiences of treatment procedures are framed in a much less intrusive
and overwhelming way compared to women who enter into treatment with the
purpose of having a child of their own. Specifically, through cluster analysis,
bodily experiences is examined through the physical (injection pain; side effects),
emotional (stress; sadness), and cognitive (attention, distraction) variables (2017,
p. 25). Survey findings show that IVF patients and egg donors report of similar
physical pain but that IVF patients experience a more intense bodily experience in
finding the treatment process much more draining emotionally and cognitively.
The discernible dissimilarity is ascribed to the different reasons for undergoing
treatment and shows how the motivational factors affect the bodily experiences of
IVF. Consequently, they argue, medical interventions and their effects cannot be
approached in a universal fashion – nor can biology – but variation needs to be
taken into account in a systematic way (Almeling and Willey, 2017).

The interlinkage between motivational factors and bodily experiences of assisted reproductive technology illustrate how the technological and socio-cultural interacts. As Bauchspies et al. summarize:

> Technology is part of the context and shapes the interactions of participants in a social situation when actors interpret the meaning and affordances of a technology and act with it.
> –Bauchspies et al. (2006, p. 85)

Hence, it provides a case in point for a contextualized and situated approach to reproductive technologies as argued by Haraway (see Chapter 2) and for taking into account the lived experience of assisted reproduction as expressing a dialectic process in the technologies shaping and being shaped by cultural and individual forces as described by way of introduction. The specific interrelations between technology, motivations, emotional, cognitive and physical impacts shown in the findings above, also illustrate the duality between discourse and materiality in its specific knotting together of socio-cultural discourse and biological materiality with the techno-scientific intervention of reproductive technologies (Haraway, 2004a).

The techno-social point of context is particularly supported in this study' research findings in terms of the general tendency for the women to alter their perceptions of the technology during treatment processes and to continuously negotiate acceptable boundaries for treatment while also drawing on existing cultural knowledges, practices and norms. In this regard, they consequently negotiate ideas about 'natural' and 'normal' conceptualizations and while their actions are influenced by applying the technology, many also question and challenge specific procedures, for instance in regard to hormone treatment as particularly expressed in Marie Louise's narrative above.

5.4 Reworking Boundaries of 'Natural' Processes

> You move your boundaries all the time, because you just want to have this child.
> –Thilde (Nurse, 3 month-old son through IVF/ICSI)

The quotation by Thilde very much captures the essence of why undergoing fertility treatment is also often a process of re-working one's initial boundaries, conceptions and expectations. As described in the previous chapter, the self-projection of motherhood remains an identifying point of reference throughout the women's biographical narratives and the biographical revisions made – including the decision to embark upon medically assisted reproduction – are always centred around the desire to have a child of one's own. As with the decision to embark upon solo motherhood, moving one's boundaries in the treatment process can also be viewed as a continuous response to changed circumstances and contexts and new options/limitations present. Coupled with 'the open ended' nature of treatment and, as reflected in Cecilie's and Anne's narratives above, a growing knowledge about working procedures and indicators for positive outcomes (regarding the quality, number and size of eggs for instance), they continuously assess and interpret presumed likelihoods for success against risk factors and the physical and emotional consequences they experience or expect to face at some point. In these assessments lie also considerations about how the 'conveyer-belt life' of treatment (Christina) will influence their life more generally. This could be in regard to their work life, social relations or for the women who already have children, concerns about how treatment may affect them.

Four of the women who are pregnant or have become mothers through IUI state that they do not believe they would have continued with IVF treatment had their IUI treatments been unsuccessful. Others, such as Ditte, tell of being close to terminating IVF treatment:

> I'd had the first attempt just before, directly after the treatment, and that didn't work, and then there was one egg left and she is lying in the room next to us. And I'd already decided that that would be the last one, because by then I'd used so many years on it, and so much money and I just couldn't face it any more. I might have given it one more try if it had fitted into my programme, but I was just so tired because it's incredibly tiring, and people that go through seven IVF treatment, uh, I can't imagine what that must be like, it must be really hard, so I think I've been really really lucky.
>
> –Ditte (Lawyer, daughter age 1 through ICSI)

For others who have experienced a number of unsuccessful rounds of IUI treatment, moving on to IVF treatment was seen as a positive move that gave renewed hope for success as Cecilie describes in her introductory narrative. Due to the many different and complex considerations mentioned above, the women express various attitudes towards treatment continuation and termination. Tina describes it in the following way:

> When you make a decision like this, you do what you have to. It's just what you do. [...] Then you can kind of, you know, you have a journey, where you say, well we'll start here and then I've got this possibility and this possibility. I just never got so far. That's where I think you'll hear that people experience completely different thoughts, because if you don't experience it for yourself, you can't really imagine what the next step will be like.
>
> –Tina (Business manager, 5-month-old daughter through IUI-D)

It is impossible to know whether the women who experienced successful treatments would have stopped treatment before IVF had they not become pregnant. The sample also only includes women in treatment and not women who have terminated treatment. When taking these reservations into account, when comparing prospective and in particular retrospective reflections on treatment, a general tendency to move on to a next phase of treatment can be seen if the current form of treatment proves unsuccessful. Based on her experiences as a nurse in the fertility clinic at Rigshospitalet and her work in the network groups for solo mothers, Maria Salomon observes a similar tendency. She describes the decision to embark upon IVF as a decision that often has to 'mature', for instance during a number of unsuccessful IUI treatments, after which many become ready to move on to a next phase of treatment (Salomon, expert interview).

As described previously, I find this kind of boundary-work to be closely interlinked with the theme of re-defining and re-negotiating perceptions of 'natural' processes. In this regard, Karoline provides the following reflections on moving one's boundaries in the quest for a child:

> Well I think because really early on I worked with my body and who I am, I could feel very clearly that biologically and emotionally, that it should be my child. Full stop! *Laughs* Well, that's the first wish, and then I take things like, it's just something that I can feel biologically and emotionally. If at some point, maybe in a year or two, I find out that it's unrealistic, then my…my boundaries might move, I know now, I don't know how, but if they then say 'Now there aren't any more good eggs, now you have to buy eggs abroad' for example, I know that I wouldn't want to do that, that would be my limit – but ask me in two years' time! It's possible that it'll change. I'm really like, that our identities and the whole thing changes in relation to context and suchlike, completely. So, that's what I would answer right now.
> –Karoline (Artist, in treatment with IVF)

Besides pointing to the processual nature of identification, Karoline illustrates how the wish for an own child interrelates with understandings of 'natural' processes that may transform concurrently with the options of treatment available. For instance, if IUI does not work, the next likely step will be IVF. If IVF proves unsuccessful, some may start to contemplate the option of double donation or adoption. These contemplations open up the discussion of the importance of social and bio-genetic aspects of kinship and the strategies of 'strategic naturalization' used to claim an own child as a single woman embarking upon solo motherhood. Given that these aspects will be discussed in the next chapter, I will merely add here that the common and initial wish to stay as close to the 'natural' process of procreation as possible also interrelates with a number of other issues, such as the wish to stay within the limits of one's own 'biological' fertility and to avoid the risks and emotional upheavals potentially associated with hormone stimulation. The boundary-work performed in the process is sometimes a matter of setting aside ideas about 'natural' procreation because the wish for an own child becomes more important. Most often, however, their narratives suggest that these ideas and conceptions are re-defined during the process whilst the technologies themselves are concurrently perceived as more 'naturalized' and ideas about ideal family formations and the social and biological aspect of kinship are reworked.

5.4.1 (Un)manageable Bodies: Performing Biological Responsibility

While the fear of 'not knowing' the outcome of the fertility process causes emotional distress, I have also argued above that the physical and emotional strain reinforce each other. The stress of 'not knowing' incorporates concerns about how the women's bodies will react to treatment. It is evident from the individual narratives that their experiences of undergoing different procedures of fertility treatment emanate from the bodily experiences of treatment, because these are in focus throughout treatment. Considerations such as whether diagnosed or potential fertility issues may influence the process, concerns about their 'biological' age, how they will respond to types and amounts of hormone treatment, how many eggs they are going to produce, the quality of them and the success of fertilization are examples of ongoing reflections that also add to concerns about how the body is going to perform.

While these bodily processes are increasingly seen through the means of technology, the women in this study do not see reproductive technologies as a 'quick fix'. As Ditte states:

> ... I say to people who wait, because yes, you can always just get fertility treatment, but it's not a magic wand! It's just not a magic wand! There's still so much they can't control.
> –Ditte (Lawyer, daughter age 1 through ICSI)

This is not only with a view to technological advances but equally in terms of regarding the body as a living fact that remains outside individual, discursive and techno-scientific control. As Christina for instance narrates:

> It's such an individual thing, how people respond to [hormone treatment], and it was really a difficult thing that whenever they made a decision about something, 'your body's going to do this', then my body went and did the complete opposite! So my hormone treatment was turned up and down and at points it was like I could feel my ovaries on the outside; my mood went up and down.
> –Christina (Social worker, in treatment with IVF)

The 'unmanageable' aspect of how bodies will react to the treatment procedures speaks to the 'agency of bodily matter' (Haraway, 2004a; Lykke, 2010) and to the interdependence of both techno-cultural discourse and biological materiality in the process (Haraway, 2004a, p. 67). Hence, when we are to understand how emotional and physical processes interlink and reinforce each other, the stress related to unknown bodily treatment responses constitutes an important factor. At the same time, efforts are made to manage bodies through techno-cultural discourses, and through individual measures performed as well. This relates to the time-tabled and 'interval-living' nature of treatment and to considerations about diet, exercise and so forth.

> As knowledges and beliefs about one's biological and genetic complement become integrated into the complex choices that prudent individuals are obliged to make in their life strategies, biological identity generates biological responsibility.
>
> > –Rose (2001, p. 19)

In terms of 'managing' one's body in the fertility treatment process, the concept of 'biological responsibility' (Rose, 2001, p. 19) proves illustrative. Throughout the treatment process, the women take part in many decisions regarding their treatment, for instance regarding the number of embryos to be transferred:

> So then they asked, did I want to have them both put in, with the risk that they might turn out to be twins. Of course, even having one put in might result in twins, but the risk is a bit higher with two. And they said that that's what they would recommend, seeing how it was a one two-cell and one four-cell. So if I were to only have one put in, then naturally they'd go for the four-cell.
>
> > –Anne (see narrative above)

While the individual and 'biological responsibility' performed may add to a greater exercising of agency in the process, it may also increase one's sense of being responsible for unsuccessful rounds of treatments and possibly add to the emotional distress. In terms of exercising agency, I previously described how the women seem to adopt a more instrumental approach as treatment progresses and they become more familiar with treatment procedures. This seems to both increase one's agency regarding navigating within the system and the resources available, while also adding to the gradual embodiment of the particular doxa (Bourdieu & Wacquant, 1996) characterizing the field of fertility treatment. It also relates to the number of ontological transformations that take place during the course of treatment and likewise to the interplay of technological objectification and individual agency inherent in the 'ontological choreography' performed (Thompson, 2005). For instance, states of feeling objectified or alienated occur at times and come across in the narratives in statements such as feeling 'disconnected' (Thilde), feeling like a 'guinea pig' (Christina), of losing one's 'privacy' (Maria) among other similar statements. The timetable regime of hormone treatment for example, as well as the experiences of discouragement seem to add to this state. However, as Thompson (Cussins) shows (reproduced from Chapter 2):

> The women's objectification involves her active participation, and is managed by herself as crucially as it is by the practitioners, procedures and instruments. The trails of activity wrought in the treatment setting are not only not incompatible with objectification, but they sometimes require periods of objectification.
>
> –Cussins (1996, p. 580)

The active participation of the women in their treatment procedures, of entering into dialogue with the clinical staff and of sometimes challenging recommendations add to the exercising of agency during the process. In addition to this, the increasingly instrumental approach to treatment points to the active participation of managing one's body as an instrument in which the women are also able to 'enact their subjectivity through their objectification' (Cussins, 1996, p. 576).

5.4.2 Attitudes towards the Technological Possibilities of Assisted Conception

In the introduction to this book, I included the paradoxical tension which reproductive technologies pose for feminists. On the one hand, they may help to alleviate the distress of infertility while at the same time potentially adding to the gendered expectations of reproduction, thereby further increasing the distress of infertility (Thompson, 2005). In the interviews, the women first and foremost highlight the positive aspect of having access to and being able to apply the technologies. They do not experience an increased pressure to use them now that they are available; instead they are primarily seen as a means of providing a morally responsible route to motherhood as well as of improving their reproductive choices. The technologies are perceived as empowering rather than suppressive. While the women do not question the fact that they are also part of a biomedical industry and a greater 'machine', it seems as if the equal access to publicly funded treatment, as well as to general welfare state services such as day care, child benefits etc. reduce power inequalities by making medically assisted reproduction a less stratified option (see Chapter 4). Furthermore, the general prevalence of reproductive technologies with 10.5% of children born in a given year being conceived via assisted reproduction (see introduction) and likewise the increasing normalization of the technologies, presumably add to the women's view of reproductive technologies primarily as a positive resource. The discursive change of terminology from *artificial* insemination to *assisted* reproduction implemented in legislative Acts from 2013 symbolically substantiates the process of normalization within this area of reproduction.

The more negative aspects of medically assisted reproduction gaining currency are primarily related to the following three issues in the narratives: Firstly, the prevalence of the technologies could potentially add to an individualized culture that may further complicate the meeting of a partner, as discussed in the previous chapter. Secondly, in addition, some women mention that they would be against gender selection, in popular terms also referred to as 'designer babies', and that this would be extending the possibilities of the technologies too far. As with most countries, gender selection is not permitted in Denmark. Thirdly, two interviewees mention that some might feel pressured to use medically assisted reproduction due to societal expectations of motherhood.

While the interviewed women primarily frame assisted reproduction as a way to fulfil their wish of an own child and as a means through which to realize their revised life plans, the paradox remains. On the one hand, the normalization of the technologies may positively add to the growing acceptance of 'new family' forms such as the solo mother family, and may figure into a socio-cultural context characterized by other social transformations such as general changes in family demographics and the production of new legislation. On the other hand, throughout this book, I demonstrate the distinct ways in which the women also 'build on existing cultural models' (Becker, 2000, p. 35). In the next chapter, I will show how the strategy of naturalizing the bio-genetic link between motherhood and womanhood serves as a way to legitimize their particular route to motherhood. Paradoxically, while extending the notion of motherhood it may simultaneously reproduce its cultural significance. By means of the technologies, it may furthermore add to the 'culture of perseverance' (Thompson, 2005, pp. 94–95) and to the emotional and physical distress of undergoing treatment.

In this chapter I have explored the lived realities of undergoing fertility treatment and examined how these experiences are shaped by the relationship between socio-cultural discourse and biological materiality on the one hand and the techno-scientific intervention of reproductive technologies on the other. I show how the technologies are mainly perceived as a positive resource for reproductive assistance and seen as a possibility to pursue a morally responsible route to solo motherhood. In detailing how the women in this study conceive of and engage in assisted reproduction, I expand on the argument that moving and re-defining one's boundaries of ideal and natural processes in the quest for a child is closely inter-linked to the process of undergoing fertility treatment. For instance, when comparing prospective and retrospective reflections on treatment procedures, I generally find a tendency among the women to want to embark upon treatment that resembles 'natural' processes of procreation to the extent that this is possible and for a number of interrelated reasons. Furthermore, if the form of treatment they are undergoing proves unsuccessful, I see a tendency to want to move on to a next phase of treatment as a response to changed circumstances and contexts.

The women's narratives on undergoing fertility treatment also show that the process is often characterized as a 'emotional roller-coaster' (Thompson, 2005, p. 93) due to experiencing alternating states of hope and discouragement that are closely interlinked with the fear that treatment may not result in pregnancy and motherhood. In this regard the chapter explores the physical and emotional strain of undergoing fertility treatment and the ways in which they interlink and reinforce each other. While the stress of 'not knowing' primarily causes emotional distress, it is also embodied in concerns over how (un)manageable bodies can be managed and can perform in order to improve one's chances of successful treatment.

Chapter 6

Forming Donor-Conceived Families: The Complex Interplay of Biogenetic and Social Ties

Genes and environment are mutually interdependent throughout life trajectories, 'shaped by the interplay of specificity and plasticity', which according to Steven Rose leaves the dichotomy between nature and nurture 'spurious' (1997, p. 306). Mukherjee phrases it more bluntly:

> It is nonsense to speak about "nature" or "nurture" in absolutes or abstracts. Whether nature – (i.e. the gene) – or nurture (i.e. the environment) – dominates in the development of a feature or function depends, acutely, on the individual feature and the context. (2017, p. 481)

While the 'gene's-eye-view' of the world (Rose, 1997, p. 6) have lost some of its distinctness and the social and medical problem-solving-potential of genetic research has been rationalized, the 'geneticisation of society' still very much influence our understanding of, and thinking on, individual behaviour and personality. Kinship, too, in terms of the importance of genetic links, proper gene pools and knowledge of one's genetic inheritance seem to dominate our thinking on the formation of kinship and family (Nordqvist and Smart, 2014, pp. 144ff; Nordqvist, 2017; Hertz and Nelson, 2019, p. 5).

This chapter explores the question of to what extent genetic understandings of kinship influence the way in which the interviewed women reflect on and negotiate kinship as both an imagined and lived practice. I explore how the women in this study conceive, conceptualize and enact the notions of family and kinship in terms of creating significant relations and networks. Furthermore, I discuss how a complex interplay of biogenetic and social ties impacts on these family conceptions, and how these are shaped within ideal expectations and family practices experienced, as well as within chosen life plans and life chances available. Hence, the underlying argument in this chapter is that the importance attached to both biogenetic and social origins, is shaped by different kinds of personal biographical experiences in terms of the interviewees' own upbringing, line of employment and other biographical factors.

Lived Realities of Solo Motherhood, Donor Conception
and Medically Assisted Reproduction, 127–160
Copyright © 2021 Tine Ravn
Published under exclusive licence by Emerald Publishing Limited
doi:10.1108/978-1-83909-115-520211008

Furthermore, the chapter operates from the underlying argument that the perceived and attached importance of biogenetics and social origins is also influenced by the fertility treatment process itself, as well as by dominating cultural narratives about procreation and family formation. This speaks to the greater theme of integrating the reciprocity between individuals, society and technology in order to understand, in this chapter, the lived experiences of relatedness from the perspective of single women embarking upon solo motherhood. Yet, the key issue is to make visible the complex and multifaceted 'choreography between the natural and cultural' (Thompson, 2005, p. 177) employed in the recognition and negotiation of relatedness. Hence, a main objective is to elucidate the transformative processes and biographical particulars when drawing upon, negotiating and transforming specific and dominating socio-cultural narratives. In this regard, the concept of 'choreography' lends analytical power to the exploration of the particular ways the women in this study 'do' and (re)define kinship both as an everyday and an imagined practice based on certain personal and culturally shaped ideals about doing family.

6.1 Three Biographical Narratives on 'Having an Own Child'

Below, three different presentations and analysis portraying three diverse and condensed biographical narratives have been composed to illustrate the importance attached to 'having an own child' (Lesnik-Oberstein, 2008) in the full biogenetic sense. Each presentation includes relevant biographical data and key narratives and seeks to illustrate the diversity, similarity and complexity of the accounts. In chorus, these three biographical narratives act as small exemplary cases and as a lens through which to further explore the main and shared themes that figure across the entire set of life story narratives.

6.1.1 Christina

At the time of the interview, Christina is a 32-year-old woman who lives in a medium-sized city in the central part of Denmark and she works as a social worker. She grew up with her parents and a younger brother. The man she refers to as her dad is not her biological father, but he adopted her when she was a child. She has recently made contact with her biological father but she only briefly mentions this in a closing comment when talking about factual data. Christina has been diagnosed with PCO (PolyCystic Ovaries), a condition that can cause irregular ovulation as it did in Christina's case. She was told that it was unlikely that she would ever be able to have children and she initially considered adoption due to her strong desire to become a mother. Eventually, however, she began to have regular periods and was subsequently told that with the right kind of treatment, she would have a chance of becoming pregnant.

After that, I dropped the idea of adoption because I really wanted to carry a child myself. And for me there's something special about the idea of carrying a child for nine months - and the bond that's created – compared with adopting a child. But I've never ruled out adoption and I would still consider it if the other way [fertility treatment] doesn't work out. On the other hand, if you're single and apply for adoption, that's when it can really take many years. My parents know someone who's done it, and it's taken nearly 7 years for her case to be processed – from when she started to...and that's just really crazy. With adoption, you're not given equal status, you're not treated the same as when a couple applies...and then there's also the issue about the children you adopt, that there are other things involved that mean that they often have some challenges...Yeah...I think that was pretty much my decision about going with a donor being the path I wanted to take.

Christina originally begins fertility treatment with her former partner. Initially, he is not interested in having more children, but then changes his mind. From Christina's perspective however, he is never particularly involved in the fertility treatment process, and when he proposes to her on her 30th birthday, she declines. Following this turning point and a subsequent period of dating, having not met a potential partner, she decides to embark upon solo motherhood. She is not daunted by the thought of doing it alone, having also seen how well her own mother managed as a single mother when she left Christina's biological father. Christina then decides, in her own words, to 'take responsibility for my own life and decide for myself...'. The decision marks a transformative event in her life and acts as an internally driven catalyst for redirecting her biography. In general, the plot line in Christina's account is structured around the issue of claiming agency and independently creating new meaning structures in her life by explicitly challenging the standardisation and normalisation inherent in the 'normal biography' and in the nuclear family ideal. Exercising independence and strength also come across as a theme when Christina talks about having to make hard decisions and cope with very difficult experiences.

Following the decision to embark upon solo motherhood, Christina starts treatment and after an arduous process of hormone regulation, becomes pregnant. When she is 20 weeks pregnant, doctors discover that her baby has a severe cleft palate and ask her to consider a late-term abortion. Considering the life her son would have with 21 operations within the first 1.5 year of his life, she applies for an abortion. However, her application is declined as she is deemed resourceful enough to have the child. The doctors then offer her a genetic test and on the morning she attends the hospital for the test, her son dies. After a process of recovering from the loss of her child, she begins IVF treatment again with the use of a non-contactable donor/anonymous donor. The second round of treatment does not however, result in pregnancy. She then takes a break from treatment, due among other things, to a change of job. At the time of the interview, she is ready to initiate a third round of IVF treatment.

In elaborating on the importance of nurture vis-à-vis nature and her considerations about donor insemination, Christina narrates the following,

> Thinking about my own decision, I think that I've had a mother who was able to do things on her own, who has shown me that it could be done, even nearly 33 years ago... Life was different then and she was alone with me - my grandmother helped of course - but it made me think, I can do it too! She lived in an apartment and only had a bike, and I live in a house and have a car – of course I can do it! And it also made me think that I've got some power in me, both something genetic but also – yeah – that I've never really doubted that I could do it. Then I also think that after what I've been through – I've also considered whether I have with me some genes which make something in me work against a pregnancy or that aren't good. On the other hand, I do believe that I have something good to pass on, because I've had that myself, but that was both via genetics and environment since my dad is not my real dad, and he's had a huge influence on the person I am today. And that's how social inheritance comes to be a part of who you are. And that will be the same for my child, since my child won't have a father, but in that sense, I'll be able to give him with some social inheritance in a good way ... in relation to other men...'

When asked directly about the importance of having a biological child of one's own, Christina states that this is her 'first priority' in terms of 'being able to carry on one's genetics' and that there is something significant in the fact that one's own body has helped to create the child. However, Christina sees other routes to motherhood as possible as well, and states that she would not be worried about considering egg donation (which in her case would be a double donation) and refers to a friend who has chosen this route. Asked directly, she states that she would probably prioritize egg donation before adoption, because egg donation would allow her to carry out a pregnancy. She continues by stating that from her job, she knows the importance of mother-child relations established during pregnancy, not only in terms of attachment but also in terms of the development of parental skills. With regard to passing on genes, she considers herself to share what she believes to be a common curiosity about parent/child resemblance in the genetic sense. 'I wonder what my child is going to look like; what it will get from me and what it will not'. She once again mentions the perspective of 'passing oneself on' genetically, but also says that the matter of genetics is not so important as to make other routes to motherhood categorically unimaginable, should they turn out to be necessary in order to have a child. With donor insemination, however, the genetic dimension is allowed to remain an important factor.

6.1.2 Anna

Anna, 40, is an associate professor. She has a four-year-old daughter with her ex-husband, who she divorced when their daughter was 2-years-old. She has always travelled and worked all over the world. Her parents divorced when she was younger and her biological father died when she was 6 years old. At this age, her mother met Anna's stepfather with whom she subsequently had two children, Anna's two younger brothers. Anna had always wanted another child and a younger sibling for her daughter and does so still, and has therefore decided to initiate fertility treatment on her own following the divorce. Considering how easily she became pregnant with her daughter in her mid-thirties, she expected a swift second pregnancy, but after going through five rounds of donor insemination (IUI-D) and three rounds of IVF treatment at a private clinic (three times with fresh embryo transfer and three times with frozen embryo transfer (FER)), she has yet to become pregnant. For all rounds of treatment, except one, she used a contactable donor/open donor. At the time of the interview, she has decided to continue with IVF treatment in the States, and is considering the possibility of embryo donation/adoption.[1]

Beginning her narration, Anna gives special initial narrative emphasis to her life with her ex-husband and the now very strained relationship she has with him. The implications of this relationship run as a general plot line through her narrative, and influences her current life plans and biographical revisions. Furthermore, with regard to the theme of having a child of her own, she presents another meaning of 'one's own',

> He [ex-husband] doesn't talk to me, we only discuss things about [our daughter], he's extreme, very minimalist, and it's very important for him to have her exactly half the time even when it doesn't suit her, and then she tells me that she doesn't want to be with daddy – it's completely ridiculous - so it also makes me feel that I want a child that no one can take away from me. One that's mine, that I have on my own. I simply can't cope with anything else, because I can't have a child with someone who would need to be involved. I can't cope with them being able to take it from me, it's just too painful to think about.

Another recurring theme throughout Anna's story is the matter of pushing one's boundaries in order to achieve the objective of having a child. This matter is very much present throughout many of the individual narratives, as well as being closely interlinked with the use of/process of medically assisted reproduction (see Chapter 5). As the following accounts from Anna illustrate, her

---

[1]Embryo adoption or embryo donation refers to 'the transfer of an embryo resulting from gametes (spermatozoa and oocytes) that did not originate from the recipient and her partner' (Zegers-Hochschild et al. (2009, p. 2685).

perception of assisted reproduction as well as her view on the importance of genetics have changed during the course of her treatment process,

> My attitude has really, really changed, back then I didn't want to have IVF because I wanted it to be natural and I didn't need this and that – and now I'm the complete opposite - now I just want a child.

In general, the theme of re-defining and re-negotiating perceptions of 'natural' processes (i.e. in terms of pro-creation, fertility treatment, motherhood, family formation, among others) represents a recurrent motif in the shared strategies used to claim a child of one's own. As will be explored through the concept of 'strategic naturalizing' (Thompson, 2005, p. 274), social and biogenetic aspects are downplayed/highlighted strategically in naturalizing some elements over others.

In reflecting on why she chose to embark upon donor insemination, Anna implicitly negotiates the importance of genetics;

> I have never ever considered adoption. I have absolutely no problem with having a child that's not genetically related to me in that sense, but I would prefer one that is genetically mine. I love being pregnant, it's so amazing to be able to bond with a baby, and I would like to do that again. Adoption is quite difficult and extremely expensive - at least as expensive as this [assisted reproduction] - and that's actually what has prevented me from doing it […]. It was when I was looking into prices and such like that I came across the concept of embryo donation, and then I found a Californian clinic that does it, and they have such great reviews for the whole thing. Now I'm in a Facebook group where they discuss how it works, and many of the things they say have convinced me even more. They say things like… 'I don't ever think about the fact that we're not genetically related. It's only when people say things like "she looks so much like you" that you think, no, that's impossible – but that it doesn't really matter because they're still my son or my daughter'. There was this solo mother who wrote to me, 'I was just like you, and I regret that I didn't do it [embryo donation] earlier, I have the most amazing children'. And she had this picture - these twins - and they were so adorable and then I thought, well yeah, that's also a possibility - why not? They would still be your children.

Later in the interview, when returning to the issue of egg donation, which would allow for a biological link to the child (through gestation) but not a genetic link, she again expresses her changed position on the need for a genetic connection, but at the same time she states that she has not given up on the hope of being able to use her own eggs. She hopes that an IVF clinic in the US will say that 'we have a whole different type of treatment for someone like you, your numbers are good so we believe that you will only need one round of treatment'. Then, at the time of the interview, the theme of whether or not 'to give up on passing on my genetic inheritance' is a strongly recurrent consideration in Anna's process. Following her stated hope of being able to use her own eggs, she also narrates,

> I want it to happen, but at the same time there is this cloud hanging over me of just wanting a child. I just want a child. It comes and goes and sometimes I get quite desperate. I had this funny experience when I was in my twenties and worked in a mall in the US. My boss was around 40, and already had a child but now she had a new husband, and they were pursuing adoption and IVF. Then this pregnant woman enters and she asked for an extra favour – it was a store where we made embroidered t-shirts – and she asked about whether we could do this thing and it was a big favour, and my boss said 'yes, if you will give us your baby'. We all laughed and she left, but then my boss turned to me and said 'well you never know', and I realised she was completely serious. You never know if she had actually considered given up her baby and it was just like adoption in her eyes but it made me realise how desperate women can be when they get to that point, where they don't care how it happens, they just want a child. I've always looked down a little on people like that - I've often thought about that story - and then I end up there myself...even though I would never actually ask anyone.

At the end of the interview, when asked about what type of donor she might consider whilst in the US, she replies that the choice of donor does not matter that much anymore and that she really does not want to choose, she just wants, 'blue eyes and not too short'. Furthermore, she narrates, 'I will pass on the genes which are important'. Then at some level, I have set aside that some things are important, in the form of genetics'. She continues with the issue of genetics and says that she has considered going for a mixed race if she chooses to pursue embryo donation, because then it will be obvious that the genetic link is missing. She then concludes by saying that 'yes, genetics doesn't mean that much, it matters a lot to me to be pregnant'.

6.1.3 Marie Louise

Marie Louise, 29, is a lecturer in child psychology/pedagogy. At the time of the interview she is six weeks pregnant after her first round of treatment with donor insemination (IUI-D). When she is asked to tell her life story from the time she finished lower secondary school, she begins her narration by stating,

> In order to give you the whole story, I'll begin before I finished lower secondary school, because some very significant events

happened in my life, about which I am very reflective and balanced today, but which really influence who I am. When I was seven years old, my mother died in a car accident and after that I lived with my dad who is brain-damaged. We had some help so that every day things could function at home – there were five children in my family. When I was ten years-old, I went to live with my aunt and uncle, and they become my foster parents until I was 18. They've helped me with pretty much the whole process of personal formation. There wasn't much of that before, apart from the many loving childhood years up until I turned seven and my mum died.

The death of Marie Louise's mother, and her move to live with her aunt and uncle, mark major and essential turning points in her life story and do, in more or less implicit ways, structure her narration. In this regard, the plot of nature vis-a-vis nurture is very much present throughout her narrative account. According to Marie Louise, her experiences, education and reflections regarding the importance of social and biological inheritance have been of great importance in her choice of donor insemination as a road to motherhood and to her decision to use a contactable donor/open donor. Speaking about the donor, she remarks that she has also reserved five straws of donor sperm for a second child by the same donor, which would make the children genetically related.

As part of her main (and uninterrupted) narration, Marie Louise narrates the following regarding reflecting on the choice of donor:

> [I] have very much concerned myself with genetics and personality development, what is genetic and what is environmental, especially since - as a result of my upbringing - I know how important the social setting has been, and can also see in the difference between me and my siblings, how important the social setting has been. My two younger sisters have been in foster care and my two older siblings have taken care of themselves, so I can clearly see the significance of environment. It really made a positive difference for me that my aunt and uncle took me in, they really helped form me, they gave me some cultural codes and some capital, which I've been able to use to get me through further education, and have taken into my adult life in general. I wouldn't have had any of that if I'd stayed at home. So yes, environment matters, a lot. I'm a social psychologist at heart, but [biological] inheritance and genetics are important too, because there are some things that are just hereditary, that's been established.

In her life story narrative, the theme of making the most out of the life chances given is linked to the 'painful awareness of the fact that love can be taken from you and people can leave you'. At the end of the interview, she returns to this theme by saying that;

I have always known that one is alone and that one has a responsibility, maybe I've also had a heart-rending awareness of it, but I have always taken on that responsibility because I have an enormous need for a sense of security, of knowing that I can take care of myself.

When asked to specify what it means to have a biological child of one's own, she replies,

Well, it means almost everything. Because I don't want to adopt, I won't. (...) I have some rather clear experiences from my own life about the significance of primary relations, birth and inheritance, and I don't want to...when I have the possibility of giving birth and creating a safe biological bond from the outset, as happens when you give birth, then that is my strong preference. (...). It would really have meant such a lot to me to have known my own biological inheritance, but instead I have a mother who died when I was only seven, right? There are things that I remember about her, which I'm so glad about because it also provides me with a way to understand myself.

Additionally, when asked about her reasons for undertaking donor insemination, she narrates that,

I wanted my own children, wanted to give birth to my own children, it was very important to me. I was present at my sister's first birth, and he came out with his head turned towards me, with the father sitting on the other side, and I believed that he has looked in my direction ever since, and he does, he adores me and I adore him, and we have a very special relationship, and that kind of attachment at a birth and... To be pregnant carrying around a big cumbersome belly, I have never been in doubt about wanting to do that so I haven't considered adoption at all.

She did consider the model of a 'rainbow family', partly because that would allow for the presence of a biological father in her child's life, and she finds it awful that two men who love each other cannot have a child together. She abandoned this possibility because she did not know of any potential candidates and she was not interested in the potential complications such a constellation could bring about.

6.2 The Complex Interplay of Biogenetic and Social Ties

The issue of nature vis-à-vis nurture is very much present in the three afore-mentioned life story narratives. It is evident that all three women find both the biogenetic and social aspects of kinship and inheritance important in their pursuit of solo motherhood by donor insemination. Nonetheless, the *way* in which the equivocal meaning of the concept of heritability (Fox Keller, 2010, p. 12) comes to matter, seems to be subject to different and changing modes of rationalization.

In the three specific presentations above, the women all use their own family backgrounds and relational experiences to establish their views on 'having an own child'. Growing up, they have all experienced close kinship relations of a non-biological character (non-biological fathers, foster parents) and they highlight these experiences in order to illustrate or support the point that the biogenetic link does not necessarily define the quality of the relationship; likewise, they emphasize such non-biological relations in such a way as to suggest that 'biological ties do not automatically translate into affinities; this requires also a sense of being emotionally connected' (May, 2015, p. 487). At the same time, for Marie Louise and Christina in particular, they strongly identify with their maternal biological inheritance; for Christina this manifests as having inherited a certain kind of 'power', whereas it for Marie Louise is manifested in the memories of her mother and the way in which she 'understands' herself accordingly. She would very much like to have known her own 'biological inheritance', as she states, and the absence of such an inheritance acts as a strong catalyst for wanting to have a child of her own that will be both biologically and genetically related to her. Her child will not grow up with his or her biological father, but due to her choice of using a contactable/open donor, she narrates, her child will have the possibility of learning about its paternal biogenetic inheritance. Furthermore, she states that

> ...as long as you do not refer to anyone as a dad or significant dad - because a child does not quite understand that – then there is no loss, there are no traumas but at a later stage, the biological and genetic interest will definitely be immense.

The theme of wanting one's 'own child' strongly intersects with the theme of choosing and relating to the donor. In Marie Louise's case, as with the other women in this study who have opted for an open donor, the primary importance is attached to the *knowledge of* one's paternal biogenetic inheritance as an essential foundation for the identity formation of the child, whereas the importance of an actual daily presence of the biological father is downplayed. The latter point is also illustrated by Christina's views on social inheritance and male influence. Such views – that there is a 'symbolic importance' of knowing and that the presence of male role models in the child's life is important, but that neither needs necessarily to rely on biogenetic relations – are also reflected in the international literature of solo motherhood (Graham, 2014; Hertz, 2002, 2006; Jadva et al., 2009a). In the next chapter, I will return to how the women in this study negotiate the role of the donor vis-à-vis a designated father.

6.2.1 Creating Attachment and Connectedness through Pregnancy

As is evident from the entire set of life story narratives, the interlinking of mother-child attachment with biology and motherhood clearly emerge, with the subtext of equating nurture with biology as a point of departure. This does not render other routes to maternity categorically impossible, but for all women in the sample, - except for one, who pursued adoption before donor insemination - the desire for their own biologically and genetically related child remains a first priority, as long as this option is perceived as possible.

This is perhaps not surprising, due to the fact that that the sample consists of women who have chosen donor insemination as a means to motherhood. What is more interesting, then, is how they themselves define and attach meaning to biological, social and genetic matters and concerns, and how their definitions are subject to constant renegotiation, redefinition and ambiguity. As mentioned, their considerations do not merely reflect the desire for their own child, they are also closely engaged with making sense of and negotiating relatedness in general. In general, the vast majority of the women point out the importance of the mother-child attachment that is created through pregnancy and infancy. As clearly illustrated by Marie Louise's narrative, such an attachment is seen as being of paramount importance, in order to secure that the child is provided with the proper care and nurture during pregnancy (through the mother's lifestyle choices etc.) and from when the child is born. Additionally, the process of carrying and giving birth to a child is also seen to reinforce the connection and bond between mother and child, thereby increasing the sense of belonging and of the child being one's 'own'. Based on the entire set of life story narratives, I find pregnancy to be the most prevalent and recurrent aspect in wanting a child of one's own. Going through a pregnancy is also closely interlinked with predominant cultural notions of motherhood and womanhood, as we will explore later in this chapter.

6.2.2 Why Donor Conception?

The use of donor conception as a means to solo motherhood constitutes the most obvious choice for most of the women in this study, as it allows them to have a child of their own and experience the process of pregnancy, gestation and birth. Nonetheless, many have carefully weighed the options available and a few have explored other possibilities before opting for donor insemination; one woman chose to pursue adoption, but found that she could not meet the legal requirements as a result of her foreign residency. She and three other women also explored the rainbow family model but did not find a suitable match. Furthermore, two of these three women also asked a friend to be the known donor. The rainbow family model and the use of a known donor would provide the child with both a biogenetic and social relationship to its father and as a result of this, several interviewees beyond the aforementioned three women find this solution suitable in theory, but have since abandoned the idea, as they either do not know a potential donor, do not wish to share their child, or anticipate a range of possible complications in terms of visitations rights, upbringing methods etc.

The wish to have an own child in the biogenetic sense is also a wish for close attachment to the child through pregnancy and infancy, which is one of the main reasons donor insemination is preferred over adoption. As seen in two of the previous life story narratives, some women never regarded adoption as an option, whereas for the majority it was seen as a second or third alternative. All women perceived the adoption route as being fraught with complications; the process was perceived as being often long, trying and expensive. Additionally, they referenced the view that single individuals and couples are not given equal status in the adoption system and outlined potential scenarios involving receiving an older and potentially emotionally neglected or challenging child. Several women explicitly state that as single parents, they would not be able to provide the proper care needed for such a child. Several women also mention the vehement Danish debate about the ethics, regulations and practices within the field of transnational adoption that have taking place and which in particular were triggered by a TV programme in 2012 called 'The Prize of Adoption'. As opposed to the UK based study on solo motherhood, in which 'many of the participants saw adoption as morally superior and more socially acceptable than motherhood through sperm donation' (Graham, 2013, p. 85), the women in this study do not articulate such a moral order between donor insemination and adoption. Critical public discourse on transnational adoption has been noticeably on the rise (Myong, 2014) and it is likely that this accounts for the difference. In retrospect, the interviewee who initiated adoption as a first priority expresses relief that she did not adopt as a result of the multitude of negative cases, saying that

> ... about saving the third world, it's nothing like that today, it's not the case that... of course you help a child, but having to take a child out of its parents arms, I simply couldn't do that. (Ditte, lawyer, daughter age 1 through ICSI)

In contrast to the issue of adoption, the interviewees in this study adopt the same position toward casual sex as a means to motherhood as in the above-mentioned study (Graham, 2013) and as in the general literature on solo motherhood (Golombok, 2015; Jadva et al., 2009a). Deceiving a man into fatherhood is primarily seen as an act of dishonesty, immorality and irresponsibility and moreover, is assessed to be highly problematic for all parties involved. Furthermore, quite apart from the risks of sexual transmitted diseases, the women are not interested in potentially having to fight with the father over parental issues and rights.

> If I'm going to do it alone, then it has to be completely alone; there shouldn't be someone who has an equal say, who has a right to see the child, and who I might end up getting into conflicts with. I don't want to create a 'divorce kid', I really don't want that [...]. And personally, I think it's better to be able to say 'I really wanted

you, so I went to the doctor and got some help' instead of saying 'well, I really wanted you so I went out and slept with some random guy'. In my opinion, it's more responsible to choose the route I've taken [...]. It's important to be able to stand by what you tell your child about how they came into the world.

–Emma (Nurse, pregnant though IUI-D)

In this, Emma represents a common position; the road to solo motherhood is seen as both a means to motherhood and as a particular type of family constellation which needs to be morally justifiable. A planned and carefully thought out process, in which no one has been exploited or deselected is indicative of a moral and responsible approach which makes the child's conception story one that is about positive and clear choices being made, rather than about the deselection or deception of a potentially random man. Hence, all the women in this study expressly state that they find it important to have made a choice that is by design and not by chance (see also Chapter 4). By constructing the choice in such a way that it can be used to legitimize the child's conception story to the child, the women also seek to minimize potential identity problems which the child may experience later on. Taking a chance with casual sex could for instance result in a situation where the father would know about the child but would not want to be involved, in which case the child's conception story would be one of deselection on the part of the father; this is not the story the interviewees want to tell their children.

The desire for one's 'own' child may be compounded by the particular biographical experiences of divorce and a complicated relationship with former partners; however considering the entire set of life stories, it also comes across more generally that a biogenetic tie to the child appears to safeguard that the child actually belongs to them and that no one can claim otherwise. Emma conveys the following, for instance:

I would never question whether the adoptive mother was the mother of the child, but it does have another mother too, well, there is also a biological mother. And with a biological child, there is only me, I am the mother in every way.

–Emma (Nurse, pregnant though IUI-D)

The maternal biogenetic link is taken to mean that the donor-conceived child is actually theirs, and in the sense of ones 'own', it remains a salient issue that no one else, including the donor, can lay claim to the child.

6.2.3 The Importance of Mother-Child Resemblance as a Basis for Identity and Belonging

Speaking about the importance of a child of one's own, several women highlight the matter of identification and being able to recognize/mirror themselves in the child. This issue of resemblance is particularly tied to physical appearance and similarity between mother and child.

> The women in my network group [...] three of them have had children [...] I don't know if they've been lucky but these babies really look like their mothers. They probably also look like their biological donor fathers, but luckily every baby shares a resemblance with their mother, which I think is really nice, and the mothers all seem to be really happy about it too [...] It's really important to them and I know it would be for me too [...]. I can feel that the physical aspect really matters.
> –Anne (Pharmaconomist, in treatment with IVF)

In addition, Mille describes:

> Well for me, I feel like it [the child] needs to be a part of me for me to be able to identify with it somehow, or so that the child can identify with us and our family; and I guess you can probably also do that when you're adopted...I'm not sure...I don't think I've given it much thought, other than this being a need of mine, that I want to, I want to be pregnant and have one that... yes... I was about to say, one that fits in, but well, my brother-in-law is half-Greenlander, so it's not like everyone is blonde and has big blue eyes, but they're still a part of our family, right? [...]. I have a need, this basic, primary human need to pass on my genes, it's difficult to pinpoint exactly what it is [...] And then it's also this desire to say 'I can do that, I've got something good to offer a child'.
> –Mille (Insurance consultant, daughter age two through IUI-D)

As Mille points out, the issue of genetics is difficult to pin down and as the former narratives illustrate, genetics is sometimes taken to be merely about passing on certain physical traits and sometimes taken to be highly intertwined with biological and social processes of attachment and identification. As Hertz writes,

> The importance of genetics is a contradictory arena from a medical perspective, particularly with regard to how much weight to give genetics in shaping lives over nurture. But from a purely social perspective, genetics is both an idea and a road map of identity.
> –Hertz (2002, p. 3)

In spite of some arguments about how to solve the nature/nurture debate in terms of determining the 'relative contribution [of genes versus environment] to the processes that makes us what we are' (2010, p. 32), Evelyn Fox Keller argues in 'The Mirage of Space between Nature and Nurture' that confusion still very much exists, both among scientists and the general public. The 'persistent belief', nicely summarized by Moore, is 'that it is possible to conclude that some traits are more genetically determined than others,' – traits such as height and hair colour - whereas in fact, it 'makes no sense to ask if nature or nurture is more important in the development of a trait, because both play essential roles' (2011, p. 2). In general, the women tend to link physical resemblance with genetic inheritance, which manifests explicitly in the choice of donor criteria (see Chapter 7). Still, they also acknowledge that both nature and nurture remain essential, but the general fluidity of these concepts and the uncertainty established about the 'relative contribution' of each in the shaping of lives, arguably contributes to the destabilisation of biogenetic facts in the individual's (re)negotiation of relatedness, and in the varying importance attached to biogenetic ties. The narrative by Marie Louise above, in which the importance of attachment at birth is linked to her special relationship with her nephew, and the comment by Anna that she alone will be responsible for passing on 'the genes which are important' are just two examples of the complex and unfixed intertwinement of biogenetic and social categories. As Nordqvist and Smart point out in their study of donor-conceived families, such intertwinements of everyday and scientific language about genetics do not reflect any misconceptions of either; rather, they reflect different metaphors and explanatory systems which are invoked to describe the complex and diverse aspects of shaping family life (2014, p. 158). As mentioned above, the use of different narratives and changes in perceptions also reflect that doing family, and more specifically, embarking upon solo motherhood through donor conception, is a process in which means and circumstances might change on the way to reaching the goal of having a child.

The aspect of passing on genes as a matter of mother-child resemblance and mutual identification feature much more prominently in the women's narratives than for example, the aspect of continuing one's genealogical bloodline and family lineage. When some of the women mention the positive family characteristics and values they wish to pass on, they primarily refer to close relatives such as parents and siblings. Again, it is as much physical likeness – 'that you can see, well, where you come from' as one of the women states, as it is 'on an emotional level... about genetics', as she also points out (Henriette, physiotherapist, pregnant through IUI-D). The matter of creating a sense of belonging and attachment to the child, then, is taken to include both a physical and emotional aspect. While the majority of interviewees explicitly state that they consider it possible to feel strongly connected to a child without there being a biogenetic relationship (e.g. in the case of adoption, in which the child still feels like your 'own' child) the sense of belonging and attachment is nonetheless considered to be made stronger by pregnancy and genetic relatedness. At the same time, genetics remains 'an idea and a road map of identity' as Hertz points out (2002, p. 3) and this aspect shines through in the narratives and in the importance attached to mother-child resemblance and mutual identification. Importantly, these aspects are generally articulated from the child's point of view:

> I would never adopt [...] I would also be worried about the kind of future the child would face, because society is just harsh, and this is

from the perspective that when you adopt, the child won't look like you. And I would find that difficult to deal with, at least as a single mother. […] in a way, as a donor child, my daughter will also be different, but she just comes from me.

–Tina (Business manager, 5 month-old daughter through IUI-D)

Tina's statement points to a very common concern among the women in this study regarding the wellbeing of their (potential) children in terms of identity issues that may arise when they grow up: The concern is whether the child will be able to identify with its peers or will experience insecurities in their sense of identity later on. Tina is one of the few to state that she would never adopt, but her quotation still reflects common perceptions on the matter. In several aspects, the quotation by Tina highlights the wish to minimize otherness for the child, and in this regard the maternal biogenetic link seems to be of additional importance, due to the absence of a biogenetic father. Her statement regarding that her child will be different but will still come from her, underlines the increased importance of the maternal genetic link, and taps into the general cultural view that identity and origins are closely interlinked (Nordqvist and Smart, 2014). Furthermore, resemblance between mother and child, as Tina also mentions, makes the genetic link more visible and, in a very tangible way, emphasizes relatedness.

All women in this study either are, or are aiming to be, the biogenetic parent to the child they have or will conceive by donor conception. While some interviewees have considered double donation, none of the women have yet done so. Anne is one of the women who considers this option, and her quotation below illustrates how genetic inheritance is seen as important for a child's identity formation. At the same time, it also shows how genetic links can be renegotiated as a basis for kinship in the process leading towards pregnancy, which is also demonstrated by Anna's narrative earlier in this chapter, and once again, the physical and emotional attachment created through pregnancy is highlighted as one strategy to assert parenthood.

To begin with, when I first starting thinking about double donation and eggs from a stranger in a foreign country, I thought… actually it was my mother who started to talk about it, and I got so annoyed in the beginning, because I just thought, I'm not ready for that at all because it wouldn't be my child. I might carry it, but I don't even know who the woman is […] and I don't know who the donor is either. It would just be some child, but then the more I've thought about it, the more I think that that's just nonsense because it would be my child. I will carry it and build a relationship with it for nine months, and then when it comes out, it's not going to be anyone's but mine, it would be my child. So I think it's been a process, a thought process, you had to… I'm certainly not as comfortable with the thought. I would prefer that it's half mine. I'm also thinking about after the child is born. 'Well, I don't know who your biological mother is, I don't know about your biological father either, but I carried you', will that be good for the child? But I'd still do it if it was my only option.

When commenting on the potential implications of double donation for the child, Anna moreover says;

> Whether the child will experience a void that can never be filled when they get older because they don't know precisely where they come from. Well, it's really positive that you can get access to the donor numbers, so that you have the possibility of potentially finding donor-siblings; so that will be an opportunity, that could give something. I think I would also feel as if I'd robbed my child of something because I can't offer them more than this, I definitely would…if I had to get eggs from a strange woman, I would definitely, 100 % choose an open donor so I could just have a little bit to offer.
>
> –Anne (Pharmaconomist, in treatment with IVF)

Anne's statement also illustrates how the maternal biogenetic link gains significance in solo mother families, where the mother will be the only social parent that the child will also be genetically related to. In turn, by double donation, the child will not have any genetic link to a social parent, and to 'compensate', a suggested strategy is to expand the genetic connections to potential donor-siblings and make sure that the child will have access to knowledge about its paternal ancestry. Still, for the women undergoing fertility treatment, the issue of double-donation is still hypothetical for most and not yet an imminent or immediately relatable option in the process towards motherhood. From a broader perspective, however, it seems to be more difficult to claim that the child will be 'one's own' as a solo mother if one is not the genetic parent to the child. As Rosanna Hertz shows in a recent study of single women pursuing double donation, the presence of a gestational link but not a genetic link to their children demand new strategies for the women as 'bricoleurs' to establish motherhood narratives and claim motherhood. For instance, new questions arise as to how they are to relate to the egg-donor and to the fact that children born with help from the same sperm and egg donor but within different families will genetically have more in common than with their (gestational) mother (Hertz, 2021).

The process of negotiating the definition and importance of a child of one's own relates to the desire for a biogenetic tie to the child as a first priority and as an aspiration to stay as close to 'the natural process' of procreation as possible. If this option however diminishes in feasibility, the perceived predominant importance of genetics diminishes too. The quotation by Anne above, and the life story narrative of Anna earlier in this chapter, clearly illustrate this process of negotiation, but the process of prioritisation is also articulated by Christina. For these women, egg donation/embryo donation is preferred over adoption, as the former allows them to carry out a pregnancy and give birth to a child, and in this way to create attachment to the child from early on. In many ways, a child of one's own connotes a biogenetic relation to the child and this corresponds with the more general perception of genetic thinking and kinship thinking being highly interconnected (Nordqvist and Smart, 2014). At the same time, the women's wish for an own child is also embedded in culturally established discourses about motherhood and parenting.

6.2.4 An Own Child as Part of Being a 'Real' Woman

The desire for an own child is also directly articulated by several women as a basic biological need; a familiar refrain from much literature on solo motherhood which sees it as a 'deep-seated need' and a 'desire to nurture' (Graham, 2014, p. 215; Mannis, 1999, p. 124). It is described as a natural force, and motherhood is conceptualized as an important part of being a 'real' woman. The following quotations illustrate the experienced interlinkage between motherhood and womanhood (Table 6.1):

Table 6.1. Quotations Illustrating the Interlinkage Between Motherhood and Womanhood.

My mother has three children and she has always told me how amazing it was to be pregnant [...] Being pregnant has always been depicted as a very big thing in a woman's life [...] To me and my family history, that experience sort of relates to being a woman.
  –Kira (Nursery teacher, pregnant with twins through IUI-D)

It's really important for me for it to be biological, but it's not that it's less right to be adopted or not to know one's biological father, but it's just important to me. Perhaps it also has something to do with femininity [...]. There's just this basic instinct in me, I am a woman, this is what I need to do [...] of course there's also something about passing on one's genes [...] of wanting to create your own family because you want to reproduce. Otherwise I wouldn't have chosen a donor who looks like me. But again, I also want to stress that I don't only want something that's just me. There's also the fascination of... I believe there's a lot that comes from nurture, too, and environment.
  –Charlotte (Physiotherapist, in treatment with IUI-D)

It's just an instinct deep within the woman, that she needs to have children, she needs to procreate and, by the way, when they're born, she needs to protect them, in a way that maybe doesn't come as naturally to the man, perhaps he's more the one, he has the hunter instinct.
  –Maria (Teacher, pregnant with her second child through IVF)

I actually think that, that thing about feeling that you're really a mother, by carrying the child for nine months. That... I wouldn't say that it was the most important part, but it was definitely something I wanted to try before I considered adoption.
  –Tanja (Export engineer, 2 month-old daughter through IUI-D)

I feel a bit like as women, we're born to be mothers. And I think when we don't get to be a mother, we're not complete.
  –Tina (Business manager, 5 month-old daughter through IUI-D)

The naturalisation of motherhood and use of more fixed social categorisations comes across clearly in this regard in the life story narratives, and the cultural norm of having an own biological child is reinforced, along with general ways in which we understand life-courses as gendered (Lock and Nguyen, 2010) in the sense that certain perceived gender expectations are related to womanhood and comprised within the female 'normal biography'.

In her pioneering work on analysing 'ontological choreography' and the dynamic coordination of the personal, political and technological as inextricably interlinked in the making of parents, Charis Thompson finds that the 'looping interaction [between 'nature and culture binaries] brings about a mixture of reproducing the same old social order and yet being something truly novel...' (2005, p. 142, see also Chapter 2). In addition, she finds that patients in the ART clinics draw on more fixed conceptualizations when practices and processes seen as natural become unstable. In this regard, 'patients and practitioners retrench into hyper conventional understandings of some of these sorting binaries to stabilize and domesticate others and remove stigma' (Thompson, 2005, p. 142). In other words, the more one deviates from culturally established norms, the greater the efforts to normalize one's situation and downplay the irregularity will be.

The biogenetic link between mother and child, in terms of attachment, nurture and of being a 'real mother' could – in line with Thompson – be argued to be of even greater importance due to the use of assisted donor conception, which then renders the more 'natural' road to procreation unstable. For instance, the particular strategy of linking maternity to biogenetic ties, and paternity to social ties in the life story narratives, could point to a wish to define themselves within well-established practices for doing family, as a way of – with a concept from Ann Phoenix - making non-normative experiences mundane (2011). The drawn demarcation of a gendered distinction between motherhood and fatherhood does not act as a devaluation of fatherhood – far from it - but instead as a means to frame maternal 'biological markers of gender' - highlighted through the importance attached to pregnancy and bodily connections - with the aim to 'normalize innovation' in the doing of kinship (Thompson, 2005, p. 143). Even though the women in this study are both the biological and genetic parent to the child or in treatment to be so, the biological aspect in terms of creating a bodily and emotional bond appear to be more significant than the genetic link, as is also illustrated by the quotations included above. This could, as Nordqvist and Smart also find in their study, account for a strategy of reducing the importance of the genetic inheritance as a way to 'manage' the genetic donation (2014, pp. 126 and 130) which in this case relates to the more or less unknown paternal inheritance. However, the symbolic knowledge of the paternal inheritance remains very important for most, as discussed earlier. In stressing the mother-child attachment created through biological processes and in the interlinking of 'real' motherhood with 'real' womanhood, the interviewees draw upon the same cultural discourses and existing gender norms that they try to renegotiate. In other words, in their 'strategic naturalizing' (Thompson, 2005, p. 274) of juxtaposing motherhood with biology, they invoke a well-established cultural identity category of women as mothers and nurturers with the aim to destabilize our prevalent social understandings of the two-parent family constellation to legitimize and expand the 'field of possibility' (Butler, 1999, p. viii) as to the doing of families.

If a Butlerian frame of reference is applied, in terms of a theory of gender performativity, the doing and sedimentation of gender (and other identity categories) can be understood as a process both contingent on and limited by prevailing discourses and regulating gender norms. In Butler's metaphor, the staging of a play requires both an existing script and individual interpretations from the performing actors (Butler, 2004, pp. 344–345; Butler, 1988, p. 526). In other words,

> …what I can do is, to a certain extent, conditioned by what is available for me to do within the culture and by what other practices are and by what practises are legitimating. (Butler, 2004, p. 345)

By amplifying the naturalness of motherhood and drawing on existing cultural gender scripts, the interviewees implicitly normalize their specific road to motherhood through donor conception in navigating within existing and legitimating practices. These practises relate to the cultural expectations of having children and to the 'proper' framework within which to have them. Hence, cultural expectations also exist for what criteria constitute 'good' mothering and a 'normal' female life course which can be related to 'normal biography' standards. Consequently, the women not only need to 'pass' (Goffman, 2009) as constructing proper families but also as claiming proper motherhood. As seen in the previous chapter, the interviewees resort to a range of strategies to do so. It was also seen that this proved more difficult for younger women embarking upon solo motherhood, as they are perceived to a greater extent as challenging the criteria for a normal female life trajectory. By re-negotiating the predominant social understanding of family formation, the interviewees nevertheless enter a complex ambit of destabilisation since the nuclear family form remains the ideal for the majority of women. The wish to stay close to the nuclear family model while praising the opportunity of solo motherhood is a general finding within the literature in this field (see Chapter 1) and it correspondingly influences the wish for an 'own' child, as Graham also argues. On the basis of her study, the desire for 'an own child' also partly relates to the wish to 'normalise their route to motherhood and to retain some elements of traditional procreation and the nuclear family they had imagined for themselves' (Graham, 2014, p. 5). In different ways then, the particular strategy of being able to claim an 'own' child as reviewed in this section, seems to be to emphasize the biological facts of life in terms of pregnancy and gestation in terms of motherhood, by means of 'strategic naturalizing' (Thompson, 2005, pp. 274–275) with the objective of normalizing and broadening the social categories of kinship relations. As Thompson argues with regard to her concept of 'ontological choreography', this does not imply that neither the biological (nature) or social (culture) are essentialized or seen as given dimensions; rather these aspects are seen as interrelated in complex ways, depending on the specific objective. In this sense, as is evident in this chapter, they are employed accordingly.

6.2.5 Five Strategies to Claim an 'Own' Child

The complex and multifaceted 'choreography between the natural and cultural' (Thompson, 2005, 177) appear in the negotiation of relatedness on the basis of both personal and socio-cultural shaped ideals about doing family. The objective of this section is to clarify the linkages between meanings attached to the notion of having an 'own' child; the main strategies applied for supporting such a claim, and the motivations expressed for reverting to these particular strategies. By doing so, the aim is furthermore to review and highlight the most salient strategies that have emerged in relation to the motivations. Taken together, these strategies can be approached as instances of 'strategic naturalizing' which epitomize how social and biogenetic aspects are downplayed/highlighted strategically in naturalizing some elements in favour of others. Based on the preceding analysis, five main strategies materialize for the ways in which interviewees negotiate the meaning of an own child:

6.2.5.1 Highlighting the Interlinkage of Biology, Motherhood and Attachment/ Nurture

The biological processes of going through pregnancy, gestation and birth are perceived as a strengthening factor in the mother-child attachment from the point of conception, while increasing the sense of belonging attached to having an 'own' child. The physical and emotional attachment created through pregnancy is seen to be the most important aspect of having an 'own' child; it is conceptualized as being as close to the 'natural' process of procreation as possible, and in this regard also serves to establish motherhood. The women's main motivation for striving to be the biological mother is not only to secure that the child actually belongs to them but also primarily to secure the wellbeing of the child from its conception.

6.2.5.2 Naturalizing the Interlinkage of Motherhood and Womanhood

Motherhood- and preferably biogenetic motherhood – is constructed as quintessential to womanhood. By naturalizing the need to have children while stressing the 'biological facts of life' in terms of procreation and associated gender norms, interviewees write themselves into culturally established discourses about motherhood and womanhood with the objective of normalizing and legitimizing their particular road to parenthood. Despite the complexity of promoting solo mother families as a 'new' type of family construction, interviewees also acknowledge a desire, through their actions, to extend the way we interpret existing scripts of 'producing' families and kinship as a society.

6.2.5.3 Relating Maternity to Biogenetic Ties and Paternity to Social Ties

A third strategy relates to the strategy of sustaining a gendered distinction between biogenetic and social parenthood. Hence, a link between maternity and biogenetic ties is highlighted, while paternity in turn, is linked to social ties. This does not imply that the significance of the paternal biogenetic inheritance is dismissed. Rather, the 'symbolic importance' of knowing one's genetic donation (Graham, 2014; Hertz, 2002; Jadva et al., 2009) is stressed by the majority of interviewees, but this biogenetic link is distinguished from the social link that a potential future and second parent will form to the child. As seen, several women draw from their own relational experiences in order to argue for the 'doing' of families and to support their view that the quality of kinship and (especially paternal) relations does not necessarily depend on biogenetic ties.

6.2.5.4 Highlighting the Importance of Mother-Child Resemblance as a Basis for Identity and Belonging

In having an 'own' child, the biogenetic tie seems to gain importance, since due to their status as solo mothers, the women will be the sole social parent which is also to be genetically connected to the child. To visualize this link, mother-child resemblance is taken by many to be of particular importance, as it is a way to reduce otherness for the child. As discussed, genetics play a significant role in the way we culturally think about kinship, origins and identity. Physical resemblance does, in a very tangible fashion, determine relatedness between mother and child and serves to underline that the child actually belongs to the mother. The wellbeing of the child in terms of reducing identity insecurities later on is crucial and the main strategy of reducing otherness for the child is deployed in several ways.

6.2.5.5 Safeguarding the Mother-Child Relation through the Biogenetic Link

The biogenetic link between mother and child seems to help ensure that the child will actually belong to them, but the need for securing an own child extends beyond this biogenetic aspect. Especially for those women who have experienced divorce and the pain and complications of having to share a child, the security of knowing that nobody else has a right to the child serves to mitigate the insecurities and vulnerabilities experienced in conflict scenarios involving other, shared children. The aspect of not wanting to share the child is also pertinent in the motivation for choosing donor insemination over for example, a known donor/rainbow family.

The five strategies seek to show the main motivations for having an 'own' child and the importance attached to both biogenetic and social origins, respectively. As illustrated by the individual life story narratives, the issue of the given and the made in negotiating kinship is shaped by the lived experiences of relatedness and other biographical particulars, and is further shaped by dominating cultural discourses on motherhood. The importance attached to both the biogenetic and social aspects of kinship is furthermore negotiable, and strategies are subject to change and modification; this seems to be particularly interlinked with the process of undergoing fertility treatment (see Chapter 5). Despite the fact that strategies and motivations may and do change in order to continually adapt choices in light of possibilities (life plans to life chances), they remain firmly anchored in the interviewees' moral convictions and desire for making what they perceive to be responsible choices for the child in terms of conception story and general well-being.

While the biogenetic aspect plays a rather significant part in the desire for an 'own' child, it is less emphasized in the interviewees' more general definition and negotiation of family and network relations. Still, a complex interplay of biogenetic and social aspects of establishing relatedness influences the way they define 'a family' compared to the way in which they actually establish them, without the two necessarily converging.

6.3 Constructing Family and Network Relations

This section discusses how the women perceive the concept of family according to social and biogenetic aspects and asks whether these perceptions have undergone change during the process of contemplating solo motherhood. Moreover, it explores the ways in which their own family histories and upbringings influence these perceptions. Finally, individual relational maps will be used to explore how interviewees actually do establish a network around the child.

6.3.1 Defining the Meaning of a Family

When the women reflect on their definition of a family, primary emphasis is unanimously placed on 'love ties', i.e. close social relations. Moreover, family is defined as something that is given for good or bad and it is often emphasized that such relations do not necessarily need to be related by blood. While terms such as 'related by blood' and 'blood ties' is by now largely replaced by terms of gene relations, within both scientific and public discourse (Nordqvist and Smart, 2014), many of the interviewees nonetheless explicitly use the concept of 'blood ties' in their reasoning; they do so not in the literal sense of inheritance, rather, they employ the term as a well-known trope or idiom to refer to ties characterized by biogenetic relations. Conceivably, this can be seen as an effort to reduce the perceived complexity of the notion of family when sorting out the meanings of it, especially since their understandings of what is given not equals biogenetic ties and is in opposition to that which is made (Carsten, 2004, p. 9). In this regard, close non-biological relations come to denote family to a greater extent than actual biogenetic ones. At the same time, biogenetic ties are still perceived as more stable and difficult to dissolve. Again, the two should not be viewed as contradictory in nature; rather, in their duality, they reflect the richness of the relatedness being formed and negotiated.

6.3.2 Maintaining, Rethinking or Contesting Existing Family Ideals?

The historian John Gillis has famously coined the term 'the families we live with' as opposed to the term 'the families we live by' to conceptualize the family relations we actually do form as opposed to the idealized ones we strive for (Gillis, 1996, p. xv). The definition of the ideal is not a static entity that remains spatiotemporally and unequivocally valid. Rather, it can be viewed as a social construct (albeit a potentially congealed one). While the women would have preferred to have children as part of a two-parent family, the women in this study hold differing and changeable views on the real versus ideal, and use different strategies to construct coherent and meaningful family narratives. As discussed in the previous chapter, the choice of embarking upon solo motherhood is imbued with complexities, and all interviewees would have preferred another family constellation. At the same time, it was also argued that the terms of plan a, b and so forth do not completely capture the lived realities of building a solo mother family, as it is very much a process in which the ideal changes in character over time. Consequently, the solo mother family constellation is embraced wholeheartedly, even though they still express a desire to find a partner eventually.

Hence, in line with other studies on solo motherhood, the two-parent family model is not contested as such but merely reworked and re-negotiated (Bock, 2000; Graham, 2012; Hertz, 2006; Jadva et al., 2009a; Mannis, 1999; Murray and Golombok, 2005a). Several interviewees explicitly state that they have had to rethink their previous conceptions of what constitutes a family. Charlotte illustrates this by stating:

> When I'm thinking family, I've also rethought what I've been used to in terms of my own upbringing. Family for me are people who are there for one another, who give support, there's intimacy, there's closeness, there's safety, it's a base. And that family, it doesn't have to be connected through genetics and blood. As I said before, well, a family can also be me meeting a man after I've had a child, and he becomes the father of my child because he forges something, he's the one who makes the packed lunches, he consoles and shows empathy, intimacy, love.
> –Charlotte (Physiotherapist, in treatment with IUI-D)

The process of rethinking family is highly intertwined with negotiating the meaning of social and biogenetic ties; to a certain extent interviewees' own upbringings, too, are held as comparative standards for how to do family. The quotation by Charlotte illustrates how initial ideals have been reworked and biographical projects consequently revised, in order to adapt to new circumstances. In general, the family narratives constructed do not come across as 'counter narratives' (Andrews et al., 2013; Chase, 2005) or as strategies of resistance; rather they appear as strategies of aligning life situations to mere standard trajectories, although with temporal dislocations.

At the same time, dominating cultural narratives on family formation are not reproduced in an unreflected manner, and while they may not be firmly resisted, they are still both implicitly and explicitly challenged and fashioned in retellings of how families can actually be formed. For instance, in responding to what a family is to her, Maria narrates:

> We have actually talked about this because sometimes our substitute grandparents are more my family than any of the others are. They are more family to me than my big brother. To me family are the ones for whom you feel love and the ones who are present; I know that my daughter and I are not the definition of a nuclear family in the eyes of others, but we are! Still, it was a bit funny because I had a bigger car, a station wagon, and then I thought 'now we're a family!' Now we have a station wagon and another child on its way, so perhaps you're not quite a family when you're two, but you're definitely a family when number three arrives.
>
> –Maria (Teacher, pregnant with her second child through IVF)

Maria's narrative both reflects the paradoxical relation between biological and non-biological relations when establishing relatedness, as well as revealing the tension between the real and the ideal in humorously both relying on and challenging the cultural narrative of the 'white picket fence'. Christina is one of the women in this study who most explicitly opts for a rewriting of the cultural narrative related to the nuclear family (cf. introductory narrative).

> I think societal values are built around the fairy tale of... and then they lived happily ever after, and they had children and bought a house and they had... well then I guess I need to rewrite that story because that is not the case, it has not brought me anything so far. So it was about me saying, this is my fairy tale, that I will go to Skive [city at where fertility clinic is located], and she had some fertility treatment and then she had a child; to make that a good story and also a happy ending, rather than...

Later in the interview, Christina elaborates on the issue of dominating cultural narratives, and she narrates:

> Sometimes I do it, too, and find myself living in a set of values according to what would look good in the eyes of others; perhaps

it's a little like that, because this is the way you acknowledge each another, you acknowledge each other according to the familiar and not so much for what is uncertain or new. I just think that our lives are so written and we are so bad at sensing whether we want this or whether we want to rewrite certain chapters [...]. Yes, what does it mean for me to become a mother? For me it's a huge gift to have a child and at the same time it's also a huge responsibility that involves a tremendous amount of love. In some ways, I think it will form part of making me a woman, and whole. You could say that wanting a child is probably a written story too, and I have considered, 'well should I'? Maybe I'm one of ones who won't. On the other hand, when I experience myself around children, I'm not in any doubt that I should, because I can see what it does to me and how happy... I also think that I have some skills to be able to do it well. I've never doubted that I should.

Christina objects to the established cultural script which, according to her, defines and standardizes 'normative life events' such as the forming of romantic partnerships and the entering into parenthood. Not only does this script structure the 'normal biography' (Hoerning, 2001), it also acts as a normalizing framework for how the script can be interpreted and for the way in which social recognition is elicited. Christina's narrative shows how individual stories are always anchored within cultural narratives: first, it illustrates how the personal and socio-cultural interrelates as a basis for identity construction. Secondly, it illustrates that meaning is individually negotiated amongst various cultural narratives (Horsdal, 2012, p. 100). With regard to the first aspect, Christina implicitly points to the interlinkage of recognition and the claiming of identity in the sense that others' (i.e. individuals, groups and society at large) external definitions/categorisations of an individual always influence the individual's own self-identification to some extent (Jenkins, 2008). Hence, recognition is a constant force in the construction of a coherent sense of identity (Horsdal, 2012, p. 115). As the quotation by Christina suggests, this takes place in an 'internal-external dialectic of identification' (Jenkins, 2008, p. 40) and within already culturally established structures and practices. This point echoes those of Foucault and Butler, among others, who have pointed out how identity categorisations are constituted within discourses that act as frame setting for how we can 'do' and think about gender for instance, within certain socio-cultural contexts (Butler, 1999; Foucault, 1994).

Regarding the second and interrelated aspect; Christina's observation that her desire for a child is probably also a part of a 'cultural story', serves to illustrate how meaning is negotiated amongst different cultural narratives. By interlinking wanting a child with being a 'real' woman, motherhood is constructed as a more 'natural' story than that of the nuclear family, and serves as an important marker for constructing (gender) identity. Hence, even though cultural scripts are individually re-interpreted and reflect unique biographies, such as Christina's, the performative element of negotiating a meaningful subject position as a solo mother also points to common features among the interviewees' life stories. The strategy of normalizing motherhood as opposed to the two-parent family model, for example, – also described above as the strategy of 'naturalizing the interlinkage between motherhood and womanhood' - illustrates a common approach of navigating and negotiating meaning among different dominant and available cultural narratives.

A salient point here is the availability of cultural narratives. Jerome Bruner has argued that narratives not only imitate life, but that life also imitates cultural narratives (2004, p. 692). Moreover, he argues that:

> Given their constructed nature and their dependence upon the cultural conventions and language usage, life narratives obviously reflect the prevailing theories about 'possible lives' that are part of one's culture. Indeed, one important way of characterizing a culture is by the narrative models it makes available for describing the course of a life. (Bruner, 2004, p. 694)

Following this, the interviewees' negotiation of what defines a family, reflects the double-sided process in which they are both constituted and constituting themselves as subjects within existing discourses.[2] Such discourses, for example, frame how 'intelligible' (Butler, 1999, p. 22) gender can be perceived culturally. Additionally, in the process of becoming subjects, such subject positions are also challenged and negotiated (Butler, 1999). This process of navigating between established structures and exercising agency is reflected in the interviewees' particular narratives about doing and defining family. While they are in many ways at the vanguard of new kinship developments and while they cannot rely on established cultural narratives about solo motherhood, they also navigate within a 'modernist narrative of individuality', (Horsdal, 2012, p. 101), in which master narratives are increasingly challenged and in which 'the field of possibility' (Butler, 1999, p. viii) for defining 'intelligible' families has been extended. Along with variations within the 'post-familial family' (Beck-Gernsheim, 2002, see Chapter 1) come extended possibilities for identification; these extended possibilities play an important part in the interviewees' negotiations of the meaning of family.

As previously noted, several interviewees explicitly state that they have had to change their conception of what constitutes a family, and that the solo mother constellation was not what they had initially imagined. One could ask in what way their own upbringings have influenced their perceptions of family building and how this serves as a basis for identification? Is it more difficult for instance, to

---

[2]Whereas discourses comprise greater systems of thought and language that constitute the way we (partly) understand the world in outlining the field for action and meaning (Andersen, 2005, p. 51), cultural narratives comprise shared narratives at the more 'localized' level of nations and communities that assist with establishing and maintaining social norms. They can be compared to 'canonical narratives' that comprise 'normative cultural expectations' (Phoenix, 2013, p. 74) and that add to discourse practices.

deviate from the nuclear family model if one has been brought up in one? Karoline provides the following reflections on this issue:

> For me the question about male role models for the child has been of paramount importance, and this has been one of the reasons that I initially felt guilty about deselecting the man, 'can I allow myself to do that?'. And I can, because what is a father, and what was my own father? - it was my step dad, who is not the biological father, but is still just as important, or is at the same level; it is what you make of it and what you... Well, it's about making an effort to have a relationship, and I guess that if you're born into a nuclear family, then that's taken for granted. But if you've experienced since childhood, that relationships are something you do, either just emotionally and not thinking much about it, or actively and consciously, then you know that it's something you can give, and then it's actually not that problematic that exactly this figure would be missing.
>
> –Karoline (Artist, in treatment with IVF)

Moreover, Tanja states:

> I grew up having an extended family, if you will. So it's actually a natural thing for me that family is something that's not only about blood.
>
> –Tanja (Export engineer, 2 month-old daughter through IUI-D)

Despite these statements, the sample does not allow for unequivocal conclusions to be drawn between a nuclear family upbringing and the attitude towards one's own family building. In fact, 16 of the 22 women in this study grew up with both their biogenetic parents (4 of them have since lost a parent and one's parents divorced). The remaining women did not grow up with both their biological parents due to divorce, break-up or the loss of a parent. Three of those women grew up with a stepfather and two women have been partly raised in a foster family as a result of other factors.

Of course, their own experiences with specific family constellations and previous relationships, for instance, have been influential, but their perceptions of building family have been shaped by experiences that extend beyond their own upbringing in terms of next of kin. They have all been brought up in the wake of the 'second demographic transition' from the 1970s onwards, which brought for example, increasing divorce rates and a growing number of co-habiting non-married couples (Ottosen, 2005, see Chapter 1). As such, the changeable nature of family formation is part of the socio-cultural context which influences their biographical life stories. Hence, the possibility of identifying with broader cultural narratives on family diversity comes across as more significant for most as an interpretative framework for constructing meaningful family narratives. The following account from Emma recapitulates the general positioning:

Offhand, when thinking about a family, I guess it's... well the first thing I think is probably mother, father and child. But this is not what my own family is going to be like! (laughter). But I guess there are so many kinds of families, there are families with two mothers or two fathers and children, or yours and mine and ours and... Well, so this is just going to be another kind of family, where there's me and the child or children... and perhaps a man, well at some point.

–Emma (Nurse, pregnant though IUI-D)

In constructing meaningful family narratives, the two-parent family model has been rethought and re-negotiated. The nuclear family as 'the family we live by' has more or less explicitly been challenged - but not discarded - to better reflect the way family is actually being built.

6.3.3 Doing Family in Practice: Extending and Assembling Family and Network Relations

You really just create a network, and whether it's family members or close friends or good acquaintances, it actually doesn't matter; it's the network around you that's important.

–Henriette (Physiotherapist, pregnant through IUI-D)

As part of the biographical narrative interviews, the women draw a relational map and through a number of concentric circles, write down the closest and most important persons in their life. The proximity to the inner circle then reflects the closeness of the relationships. The approach of employing relational maps is inspired by Roseneil's (2006) psychosocial study of intimacy and sociability. From these maps and their narratives on family and network relations, it is evident that their children are not simply born into a small unit or dyad consisting of only mother and child, but into an extended family and broader social network, which consists of various kinds of social relations. In general, the assemblage and maintenance of relations becomes very important in building a network around themselves and their (future) children. For most, the presence and support of close relatives and friends also form an important part of their decision-making process and the subsequent process of going through fertility treatment. Regarding the assembling of close networks of family and friends, several women tell of relatives and friends who are given and enter into more significant and extensive social roles. Demarcations between kinship and other types of relations then become more fluid, as friends for instance are made into kin and in several cases are considered to be closer than biological relatives (see Franklin and McKinnon, 2001).

For instance, in responding to the question of what a family is to her, Camilla answers:

Well, it's mother, father and children, well that what it was that the first time around. As a starting point, I also grew up with mother, father and my brothers. But now I think it's ok for it to be something else. Well… what I just said about my girlfriends, that it suddenly became clear how much they mean to me. There is this saying that you can't choose your own family, but actually you can, you can agree that you want to have that kind of friendship […] where we want to be part of each other's everyday life. Yes, so for me, a family can be many things – now. The main perspective will probably still be mother, father and children, but I want that it can also be more […]. My friend for example who's married to a woman, I think it's so great that she made that choice […] She didn't expect that that was how it would turn out. And I have tremendous respect for taking - I don't know – control, but that you do what you can with your life to make it the way you want, based on the circumstances you have.
                    –Camilla (Psychologist, pregnant through IUI-D)

In addition to illustrating the process of rethinking family ideals and aligning past experiences with present conditions in order to create a meaningful and coherent life history, Camilla also offers a view of a reflective process of exercising agency within the socio-cultural narratives available, in terms of affecting the family relations that are actually formed in the sense of 'the family we live with'. In her quotation, Camilla gives the example of female friends made into kin. If we include her relational map and narratives of family and friends at large, Camilla's narrated life story illustrates most clearly the fluid boundaries between biological and non-biological relations. Camilla's relational map, see Fig. 6.1 below, shows how close friends hold the position in the inner core of her relational map and in a way constitute her closest next of kin. While Camilla's network illustrates the aspects of doing family as an exercise of choice, her told life story is also unfolded through the plot line of rebuilding her family life after her divorce and coming to terms with the grief that it turned out differently than she imagined. The constitution of Camilla's network partly reflects this duality of assembling and maintaining relations within the options available. Close relations created through her former relationship with her ex-husband have for instance been reconfigured to the extent possible and entered into new contexts. For example, the man her daughter refers to as her paternal grandfather – and who is Camilla's ex-husband's former stepfather – will also act as a grandfather for Camilla's second child.

While non-biogenetic relations may appear to be more 'given' than 'made', it is noteworthy that many interviewees apply family designations for non-biogenetic relations as a symbolic marker to express an 'appropriate' level of closeness and sense of belonging and to anchor the relationship further. Friends may for instance be designated as aunts or as sisters, and different non-biogenetic relations within or outside of the extended family may be categorized as grandparents. By using well-known idioms for kinship that traditionally are applied in Western

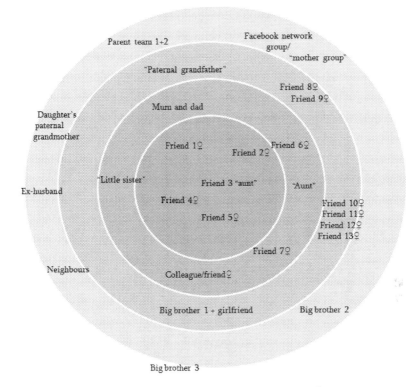

Fig. 6.1.   Camilla's Relational Map.[3]

cultures to evince a genetic relation (Nordqvist and Smart, 2014, p. 127), relatedness is re-negotiated and re-interpreted to extend the meaning of relatedness beyond the biogenetic ties. Even though familiar markers are applied, this strategy of defining relatedness substantiates the features of 'new kinship' formation in terms of emphasizing the quality of relations as a demarcation of kinship (Carsten, 2004).

The size and particular composition of Camilla's relational map does not constitute a general model for the assembling of networks among the women in this study; in fact such a model does not seem to exist, despite the fact that the majority of women include close parent and/or sibling relations in the inner core of their networks. Mette's relational map (see Fig. 6.2) and narrative account illustrates this point (see Mette's biographical narrative, Chapter 4). She lives close to her parents and her sister, her sister's husband and children. She is very close to them, sees them often, and both her sister and mother have accompanied her to fertility treatment appointments. She explicitly states that her friends are

---

[3]Specific names have been omitted from the original maps.

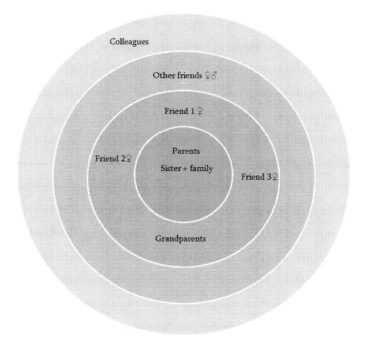

Fig. 6.2.   Mette's Relational Map.

very important to her; she has three very close friends, one of which is a single friend with whom for example, she travels and goes out. In addition, she has a large group of close male and female friends, as well as a number of colleagues with whom she also meets privately.

Like Mette, Cecilie lives close to her sister and her sister's husband and children in Copenhagen, and she has a very close relationship with them (Fig. 6.3 and see biographical narrative, Chapter 5). She sees them often and they will also assist with child care when Cecilie's son gets older. Cecilie's mother is no longer alive and Cecilie's father lives in Jutland close to the woman who Cecilie designates as her son's 'grandmother' and her husband. She considers them to be 'as close as possible to being family, without being family'. She attended antenatal classes with Cecilie a couple of times and she was also present at the birth of Cecilie's son. Besides her close family relations, Cecilie has a group of close friends, with whom she meets on a regular basis. Additionally, she often meets with friends from her network group, who include other solo mothers or women embarking upon solo motherhood.[4] Cecilie is also part of two different mother groups, one for single women, and one for both single women and women in relationships.

---

[4]The Fertility Clinic at Rigshospitalet sets up network groups for single women who sign up for fertility treatment.

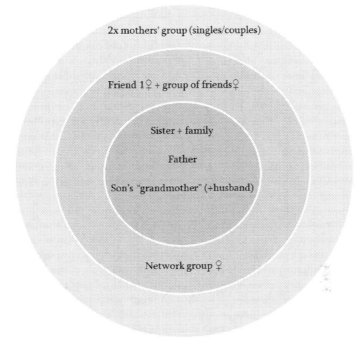

Fig. 6.3.   Cecilie's Relational Map.

The women's networks differ in size and composition as reflected by the three relational maps. The presence of 'step' and former 'in-law' relations, as well as variation in emotional and physical closeness to biogenetic parents, siblings and extended families reflect the complexity of 'doing family', and also demonstrate the more general changes in family demographics (see Chapter 1). Despite the actual size and composition of networks, and the lack of a general model, it is evident that a supportive network with close relations is mobilized on the part of all the women in this study, to the extent possible as well as to the extent required. Such a network may consist of, among others, parents and siblings, of close male and female friends who are made into kin as mentioned above, extended family relations that are reinforced, arrangements that are established with substitute grandparents, as well as involvement in physical and virtual networks with other (solo) mothers.

Managing kinship boundaries comes across as both an everyday and an imagined practice that is based on personal experiences and socio-culturally shaped ideals about doing family. In establishing solo mother families, the women both draw upon and challenge established socio-cultural narratives regarding 'proper' ways of doing family and of being a mother. In showing the interviewees' main strategies and motivations for having an 'own' child, the chapter argues that a complex 'choreography between the natural and the cultural' takes place. Moreover, by means of 'strategic naturalizing' (Thompson, 2005), social and biogenetic aspects are strategically both downplayed and highlighted in the process of negotiating and normalizing solo mother families and the wanting of an 'own' child. The strategies employed are firmly anchored in the interviewees' moral convictions but they are also subject to change and modification.

Chapter 7

Choosing and Relating to the Donor: Managing Complex Kinship Boundaries

Families with donor-conceived children – such as the solo mother families in this book – face a number of novel considerations about what constitute kin for them. How do the women, for example, view and relate to the donor in the process of selecting the donor, in the process of undergoing fertility treatment and after becoming a mother to a donor-conceived child? What type of donor do they choose, and how do they ascribe meaning to the donor connection? This chapter explores how the women in the study choose and relate to the donor as well as potential donor siblings. The genetic donation poses a paradoxical tension as it is embedded within existing kinship systems where the child and donor is bound through their genetic connection. Meanwhile, unless the donor undertakes an active role as a known donor, the donor will not participate in the child's life and upbringing, nor will they be able to form any kind of relationship with the child. This chapter sets out to understand how donors are present and positioned within solo mother families and whether donors are conceptualized as kin or as non-kin? Or if relatedness are negotiated as something in between? The distinct Danish two-way donor model that allows donors and recipients to decide the degree of openness surrounding the donation is then discussed, and the women's different rationales for choosing a certain type of donor are compared. The chapter shows that contemplations over potential identity issues figure prominently in the women's narratives, in terms of what it will mean to the children to be donor-conceived and to grow up without the presence of their biological fathers.

When single and couples embark upon donor-conception, they also enter into a web of new potential relations and connections. These webs of connections or chance network (Hertz and Nelson, 2019) constitute a novel type of network model (Frith, 2020); one which not only includes the donor, but also other potential donor siblings and their families as well. The chapter concludes by exploring how the women in this research feel about the possibility of connecting with other mothers to children with the same donor and how they regard the genetic connections shared between potential donor siblings.

Lived Realities of Solo Motherhood, Donor Conception
and Medically Assisted Reproduction, 161–175
Copyright © 2021 Tine Ravn
Published under exclusive licence by Emerald Publishing Limited
doi:10.1108/978-1-83909-115-520211009

7.1 Making Sense of Donor Relations

In their study of donor conceived families, which includes heterosexual and lesbian parents as well as grandparents of donor-conceived children, Nordqvist and Smart (2014) find the importance of genetics to be a complicated issue for the families interviewed. The issue seems to entail a paradoxical tension in the need for a constant balancing of the 'conflicting significance of nature versus nurture' in the families' renegotiation of kinship (2014, p. 150). While donor-conceived families are at the vanguard of such contemplations, as the authors also point out and as described in chapter one in this book, the doing of family and relatedness is not, and has never been, a simple or uncomplicated matter.

> Kinship is far from being simply a realm of the 'given' as opposed to the 'made'. It is, among other things, an area of life in which people invest their emotions, their creative energy, and their new imaginings.
> –Carsten (2004, p. 9)

Recalling the theoretical discussion included in Chapter 2 on new kinship theory, we saw how this 'new' approach, primarily within the field of anthropology, questioned certain assumptions which had previously been taken for granted, concerning the distinction between biological and social aspects of kinship, implicating a 'defamiliarizing' of a 'presumed natural basis of kinship' (Carsten, 2004, pp. 23 and 30). It was furthermore discussed how sketched continuities and discontinuities help answer the question of whether major changes do in fact characterize family practices experienced (Carsten, 2004; Edwards, 2009; Levine, 2008; Franklin and McKinnon, 2001). Precisely how biogenetic and social aspects of kinship inform one another and shape family practices, seems to be an enduring and recurrent question, not least due to its context-bound nature. Nonetheless, if we seek to define the characteristics of new kinship formations, Carsten highlights the explicit ways in which we define the demarcations of kinship, by various inclusive and exclusive processes. It is, after all, the 'exercising [of] choice in such a highly visible and explicit manner', that ends up capable of disrupting 'the taken for granted *quality* of the relations themselves' (Carsten, 2004, p. 180, my emphasis).

Carsten relates the increasing focus on quality not only to the private sphere but also to public and legislative debates that have revolved around for example, the right to have children. Furthermore, there are recurrent and ongoing public discussions on the consequences of new biotechnological innovations (see Chapter 3). Moreover, the exercising of choice in the designation of relations does not necessarily entail 'a highly geneticized view of kinship, where we might most expect to find it'. This point by Carsten is illustrated by the work of Monica Konrad (1998) in her study of egg-donors, in which women who donated eggs did not perceive their donation as forming one part of a future and potential genetic identity, but understood their donation of 'body parts' in a non-genetic and non-possessive fashion (Carsten, 2004, pp. 181–183). The view that the donation of eggs is primarily associated with altruism rather than financial motivation, in terms of providing a gift to help other women to become mothers, is also supported by research conducted by Rene Almeling (2009). In her study, the women donating eggs focused primarily on the future recipients, and did not identify themselves as mothers. Contrary to this finding, sperm donors are to a larger degree seen as performing a job, and the sperm donors in the study negotiated relatedness in more ambivalent terms, by recognizing and referring to themselves as being some kind of father (Almeling, 2014). Consequently, Almeling finds that biological and social parenthood act as a gendered distinction (2014). Additionally, in exploring the American market for the commodification of sperm and egg cells, she argues that,

> ...in this market, it is not just reproductive material, but visions of middle-class American femininity and masculinity, and more to the point, of motherhood and fatherhood, that are marketed and purchased.
>
> (Almeling, 2009, p. 57)

In a Danish study on sperm donation, Mohr (2015) argues that the way that donors perceive and negotiate relatedness to potential donor-offspring cannot be understood either in contractual or traditional kinship terms. Instead, the sense of responsibility and connections formed, craft a particular kind of relatedness and social significance that fall in between existing kinship categorizations.

In this study, I turn the focus to the recipients of the sperm donation to explore this complexity of relatedness and the challenging discipline of situating the donor within ordinary kinship categories. From a prosaic perspective, the donation is a financial transaction, purchased through a few click on the sperm bank's homepage and providing the receiving parties with what they need to be able to venture into parenthood. In this sense, the purchase cannot be reduced to a commercial act but must also be seen as a donation that is, as Almeling also states, emotionally charged with future visions of, in this case, motherhood. In selecting the donor, such visions are also translated into very concrete and abstract choices about 'paternal' inheritance in the bio-genetic sense. I find that the ambiguity of the donation is also mirrored in the ways, the women in this research choose and perceive the donor and that donor conceptions need to be understood in processual terms within changing contexts and life situations.

7.2 Relying on Gut Feelings: Choosing and Relating to the Donor

Donors, as Hertz has pointed out, 'have no clear place in kinship systems' (Hertz, 2002, p. 19). Does this then mean that donors are to be conceptualized and acknowledged as kin or as non-kin? Possibly the dichotomy has to be expanded with something in-between as in Mohr's study on sperms donors. Payne has termed this in-between positioning for 'un-kin' as to account for relations – for instance to those of donors – that are often characterized by equivocality in terms of clear kinship categorization (Payne, 2020).

The genetic donation from sperm donors translates into bio-genetic fatherhood, but at the same time, most donors – with the potential exception of known donors – will not be part of the child's upbringing in any pertinent sense. They will in many ways remain 'imagined fathers' (Hertz, 2002, p. 1), and are likely to be an 'absent-presence' (Zadeh et al., 2015, p. 3; Nordqvist and Smart, 2014, p. 107) at least until the child reaches adulthood.

> The genetic donation cannot be fully ignored or transcended; it is culturally coded as meaningful and inscribed within systems of kinship. This means that there is forever an underlying unresolved tension in the donor relation.
> –Nordqvist and Smart (2014, pp. 123–124)

Genetic inheritance and genetic links have gained increased significance, and our kinship thinking is increasingly intertwined with discourses of genetic inheritance. Hence, if genetic connections are strongly interlinked with notions of parenthood (Grace et al., 2008, p. 309), then how is the sperm donor conceptualized? Based on a follow-up study of 41 New Zealand couples who had used donor insemination 15–18 years earlier, Grace et al. argue that the role of the donor has changed. Typically, earlier medical practices sought to eradicate the donor as a person and negate his status as the male progenitor. The mid-1970s however, brought an increased focus on the importance of genetic inheritance as well as new and recomposed family constellations, and subsequently, the conceptualization of the donor also began to change. Along with a growing body of work on the positive effects of 'donor disclosure', i.e. of having access to information about one's paternal genetic inheritance, and political and policy measures to ensure greater donor openness, the conceptualization of the donor took on 'an entirely new and evolving profile' (Grace et al., 2008, p. 303). While many countries still only allow for anonymous sperm donation, recent years have seen the introduction of open-identity donors in countries such as the UK, New Zealand, Austria, Portugal, Germany, and Switzerland. In the Nordic countries, Sweden, Norway and Finland have also introduced legislation that make identity release donation the sole donor option (Lampic et al., 2014; Blyth and Frith, 2009, p. 177).

7.2.1 Donor Conception: Disclosure and Perceptions

Research suggests that disclosure of donor conception is less negative for children if they are told earlier in life. Those told in late adolescent or adulthood are more likely to show negative feelings towards their donor-conception, due to factors such as feeling betrayed, angry, and being denied access to medical/ genetic information, among others. Early-life disclosure, on the other hand, 'enables the information to be incorporated into the child's sense of identity' (Jadva et al., 2009b, p. 1910). In this regard, studies show that solo mothers are more likely to disclose to their children that they are donor-conceived at an early age – one more obvious reason being that solo mothers need to account for the very concrete absence of a father. However, the mother's own confidence in her choice and the method applied, based on a complex decision-making process could be another likely explanation. Solo mothers are also more likely to search for donor relations than heterosexual couples with the main reason to enhance the child's sense of identity through obtaining more knowledge about the donor and potential donor siblings as well as through potential meetings. Likewise, children born to solo mothers are also keener on wanting to find their donor compared to children born to lesbian couples. They are also more likely to refer to the donor as 'dad' and 'father' although a majority of children uses the designation 'donor' (Golombok, 2020, p. 150; Murray and Golombok, 2005a, p. 251; Hertz, 2021; Jadva et al., 2009a, 2009b). Nonetheless, literature on the perceptions of donor-conceived children remain scarce (Blake et al., 2013), particularly in relation to children in solo mother families. A small-scale US-based study comprising adolescents between the age of 12 and 17, who all had identity release donors and learned about this at a young age, reported that the majority felt comfortable with their donor-conceived status. This was particularly evident in adolescents from solo mother families, who stated that knowledge of being donor-conceived positively impacted the mother-adolescent relationship, the perception of the donor as well as the reactions of others to their DI origins. This group of adolescents also showed greater interest in obtaining information and making contact with their donors – an interest primarily explained by the lack of a relation to a second parent (Scheib et al., 2005). A study investigating how 19 children age 7–13 perceived the donor and how this perception related to their security of attachment to their mother showed that children differed in whether they had positive, negative or neutral feelings towards their donor. The study also found that children who felt a secure relationship with their mother were more likely to view the donor in a positive light as opposed to children who experienced a more insecure relationship to their mother (Zadeh et al., 2017).

7.2.2 The Danish Two-way Donor Model

Danish legislation on sperm donation was revised in 2012, to allow for freedom of choice over donation types for both recipients and donors in the medically run clinics. Prior to the amendment, medically (doctor staffed) clinics were only allowed to use anonymous sperm donation, whereas midwife (non-doctor) driven clinics, which were not part of the existing legislation, were not subject to this restriction. The 2012 amendment standardized the donation practices and rendered it possible for both donor and recipient to decide on the degree of identity-'openness' in the donation and insemination procedure, respectively. The various new donor options and guidelines were rather complex and quite opaque for recipients to navigate within (Erb, expert interview). The guidelines regarding donor choice were revised and specified in 2015. The donor options detailed in this guideline are schematically presented in Table 7.1.

The *anonymous donor* remains unknown to the recipient(s) and the child. Only information included in the basic profile is obtainable. The *known donor* is known at the time of donation and for this particular type of donation, agreements concerning paternity need to be settled prior to the donation. For the anonymous

Table 7.1. Donor Types.

Donor Type	Anonymous Donor	Open Donor	Known Donor
Donor profile information	*Basic profile*: Skin colour, hair colour, eye colour, height, weight and blood type	*Basic profile* *Extended profile*: Basic profile + for example, information about profession, hobbies, education, audio recording, baby picture	The donor is known at the time of donation
Availability of identity release information	*Non-contactable donor*: The donor is not known for the recipient at the time of donation and will remain unknown	*Non-contactable/ Non-identity release donor*: The donor is not known for the recipient at the time of donation and will remain unknown *Contactable/identity release donor*: The donor is unknown at the time of donation but the donor decides when further information can be released to the recipient and/or child. One potential model is for donors' identity to be released to the child (and the child only) when the child turns 18.	Agreements regarding co-motherhood/ paternity must be settled prior to the donation

Source: Ministry of Health (2015) (Guidelines no. 9351 of 26 May 2015).

and open sperm donation, the donor has no legal claim to paternity. The *open donor* category covers different options: (A) A donor can be open in the legal sense but remain unknown to the recipient(s) and the child. This will be the case if the single woman chooses a donor with an extended profile that remains unknown to her and the potential child. In other words, she chooses a *Non-identity release donor with an extended donor profile*. In the Danish legislation, this option is termed an open donor because all information provided beyond the basic profile is considered non-anonymous. Hence, it is possible to choose a 'non-anonymous open donor' with an extended profile whose identity remains unknown and who cannot be contacted at any point. (B) *An identity release donor with an extended profile*: Such an open donor with an extended profile will be unknown to the recipient(s) at the time of donation, but the donor can agree with the sperm bank that further information will be released at a given point. A well-known model is for the donor's identity to be released to the child only, when he/she turns 18 years old.[1] (C) *An identity release donor with a basic profile* can be chosen where only the information included in the basic profile is known to the recipient(s) at the time of donation but at where the child will be able to obtain identifying information about the donor at a given point as in option B (Ministry of Health, 2015).

The objective of the following sections is to explore how the women in this study choose and relate to the donor. The distinctive Danish legislation which includes the option of choosing either a Non-identity release or an identity release donor (in combination with basic and extended donor profiles), allows for a comparison of rationales for choosing different donor programmes, including underlying perceptions of nature vis-à-vis nurture. Other international studies have found that the donor is constructed differently based on whether they are anonymous or known (Hertz, 2002, p. 27) and that donors in particular, remain symbolically present in solo mother families (Graham, 2014). The study by Zadeh et al. (2015) supports the tendency of solo mothers to view the donor as symbolically significant in terms of being an 'absent-presence'. At the same time, among the 43 solo mothers interviewed, significant differences in how the donor is represented are exhibited. Several women for instance discursively construct the donor as an 'absence', and several women also speak of a change in their perception of the donor over time. The different donor representations apply to both anonymous and identity-release donors. Interestingly, they also find that despite the specific donor narratives created, all informants emphasize the aspects of genetic inheritance, whether this is discounted or not (2015, p. 6).

In the interviews with representatives from two of the largest public fertility clinics in Denmark, experts experience that most single women prefer an open donor, and that only a few opt for a completely anonymous donor. They find that women are divided between choosing a Non-identity or identity release donor with extended profiles within the open donor category as described above. One group wishes an identity release donor and the other group a donor with an extended profile but who cannot be contacted later on. However, the latter group still 'want a story' to tell their children (Erb, expert interview; Salomon, expert interview). In

---

[1]While this model is the most commonly known, it is not, contrary to much common perception, the only legal model of donation in Denmark. A specific time for release of documentation is arranged between the donor and the sperm bank/fertility clinic (Ministry of Health, 2015, p. 16).

keeping with other studies, such stories feature in the child's conception story and the narratives created about the bio-genetic 'father' (Graham, 2014; Hertz, 2002). These observations are supported by statistics from the international sperm bank Cryos, who has experienced a steady increase in the interest for open donors and donors with extended profiles over the last years. The sperm bank attributes the increasing demand to the growing number of single women and female couples who choose to have a child through donor-conception (Cryos International, 2019).

The women in this research have also primarily chosen an open donor and the majority have opted for an identity release donor. 15 women have chosen an open donor with whom the child can make contact at a later point (3 of these women have also used anonymous sperm donation and two women have not decided on whether to continue with an identity release or an anonymous donor). Two women have chosen a donor with an extended profile that cannot be contacted at a later point and five women have chosen an anonymous donor.

The choice of donor is made only after careful consideration of options and potential implications of the various options. One of the fertility clinic expert representatives experiences that the choice of donor constitutes a huge issue for the single women in fertility treatment (Erb, expert interview). In this regard, she points to the emphasis placed on genetic inheritance and the importance of the genetic material in terms of appearance and attributes inherited. Based on this study sample, the process of choosing the 'right' donor is, for many, a matter of careful consideration. Several interviewees describe the process as a surreal and difficult one, in which they face a number of decisions regarding the child's paternal inheritance, which they anticipate as being of importance for the child's upbringing.

7.2.3 Donor Selection and Changing Perceptions of the Donor

Almost all of the interviewees have chosen a donor with the same physical characteristics as themselves and in doing so, they adhere to the medical advice provided at fertility clinics. While some of the women explicitly point to the irregular works of genetics, choosing a donor with the same physical traits is nonetheless seen as increasing the likelihood for the child to resemble the mother. The strategy of emphasizing 'the importance of mother-child resemblance as a basis for identity and belonging' as described in the previous chapter, also constitutes a main motivating factor for donor selection. Charlotte states:

> You don't design a child. You choose something the child can identify with, with me, since I don't know if a father is going to come along [...]. Especially with looks, so that the child can identify with me. And I also believe that a lot of our personality comes from our genes. So for this reason I've chosen something close to what I can recognise. As for the decisions in general, I can't always express why I've made them because it's just been about a gut feeling.
>
> –Charlotte (Physiotherapist, in treatment with IUI-D)

Camilla describes:

> For me the most important thing is that the child shouldn't feel too
> different, you know, when things are the way they are.
> —Camilla (Psychologist, pregnant through IUI-D)

Kira adds:

> When people ask, I used to say that I looked for [a donor] who
> looked like my brothers – a male version of me and he won't be a
> completely wrong fit, right? I have this picture of a family photo
> with a bunch of tall people and then a short one. Preferably, they
> should match each other (laughs).
> —Kira (Nursery teacher, pregnant with twins through IUI-D)

Drawing on the cultural discourse of inheritance, where identity rests on the pillars of genetic knowledge, the women want to minimize the potential sense of otherness that the child might experience, if too many of its traits and characteristics cannot be traced back to the mother. One woman took a different approach and chose a donor with physical characteristics that she would have been attracted to, if she were to pick a partner. Even though resemblance in this case is interlinked with paternity, the importance attached to physical identification as a basis for the child's identity formation remains a common denominator among the donor criteria selected.

A majority of the women have chosen donors with extended profiles and therefore have access to information that can assist them with piecing together a picture of the person behind the donor number. Besides the importance assigned to the donors' phenotypical traits, many also attach great importance to the donor's values and personality. In this sense, the issue of identification is not only vital to the children but also to the mothers, and many feel the need to be able to identify with the donor. Several explicitly express that it is important for their donor to be reflective about their motivation for becoming an identity release donor, and for them to be aware of the kind of responsibility such a choice entails. Moreover, the donors' medical history also proves important for several women and it is often very specific issues that are taken into consideration. For example, if certain medical problems such as allergies or mental health issues run in the women's family, donors with similar medical histories are deselected. In general, choosing a donor is very much about finding a proper 'match' whether this is understood in terms of phenotypical traits, personal values/personality or medical history, or all of the above. Some compare the process to that of dating, although they are well aware that they are not looking for a partner or a father for their child. Still, the decision to choose the 'biological father' constitutes an emotional matter for many that often rely on a good 'gut feeling' and as with other decisions made in their process towards solo motherhood, the elements featuring in the conception story of the child need to be justified.

Justified choices do not preclude that choices can change, and choosing a donor is often a process where feelings about the donor can vary (Zadeh et al., 2015, p. 6). For some of the women in this study, access to more information about the donor also led to them experiencing a greater interest in the donor than initially expected. At the same time, several women express that the donor became less present and less important to them during the fertility treatment process. Some have to change donor(s) along the way or experience that the one they originally picked has 'sold out'. As treatment progresses without the success of a pregnancy, the wish for a child also increasingly overshadows the choice of donor. The basic phenotypical traits related to appearance remain important, but additional information becomes less so, and the donor is approached in a much more instrumental way. Anne describes the process in the following way:

> The further I am into the [treatment] process, the more... well you just sort of get desperate and think, 'I just want that child' [...]. In the end, it was more important to me that he actually had pregnancies on his CV [...]. So I thought that if I just let the biomedical laboratory technicians choose the one with the four-digit donor number who they've seen make babies before, then maybe I'll get lucky.
> –Anne (Pharmaconomist, in treatment with IVF)

Anne subsequently narrates that after having seen a programme on donor-conceived children, she is reconsidering her choice of donor and believes she will continue treatment with an identity release donor in order for the child to be able to contact the bio-genetic donor at some point. Hence, the positioning of the donor is a complex process in which the women vacillate between viewing the genetic donation as merely an instrumental means to an end, and a personalized donation. It also reflects the 'unresolved tension in the donor relation' as described above and shows that even within the treatment process, the donor is also sometimes viewed as kin and sometimes as non-kin.

7.3 Donor Relations: Coping with Kinship Tensions and Future Expectations

In addition to the donor profile criteria discussed above, the process of choosing between an identity release donor or a non-contactable donor is imbued with the same kind of tension as negotiating the donor's role in their own family formation and within the broader kinship system, as well.

7.3.1 Identity Release or Non-identity Release Donors – What Is Important and Why?

For several of the women who have selected an identity release donor, the possibility of future contact between the child and the donor was pivotal to their decision. For some, the 2012 amendment had not yet become effective at the time they initiated treatment, and in order to be able to use an identity release donor, they chose to pay for treatment at a private clinic. In arguing for this position, the women acknowledge that their children might be interested in knowing more about their paternal inheritance at some point and that it should be up to the children to make this decision and not the mothers. However, for many of the interviewees their positioning on contactable vs. non-contactable donors has not been a simple matter, and several have also changed their position prior to and during the fertility treatment process. While none of the women discount the paternal genetic inheritance and their children's potential wish to know more about the donor, many express concern that the option of contacting the donor will allow for the donor to become too strong a presence and raise false hopes as the children grow up. For some this serves as an argument for not choosing an identity release donor (see below), whereas those who have chosen this type of donor plan to mitigate potential disappointments through the donor narrative created between mother and child.

The choice between a contactable and a non-contactable donor constitutes a moral dilemma for many. The main question asked is whether it is acceptable to deny one's child a potential relationship with its paternal inheritance, despite the fact that the donor is not going to be a father and potentially does not want to take any part in the child's life. Up until the time of the interview, Mette has used an identity release donor, but she is undecided on whether to continue with this choice:

> To me it's very abstract, because it's difficult and, well, I don't have a need [to know the donor] [...] He's simply provided what was required. But of course I'm thinking about the child, and I was raised in a nuclear family with a mother and father, and I know the importance of knowing your ancestry on both sides. So of course it would be natural that the child has questions at some point, and maybe needs to know where they come from [...]. Yeah, so it's really an ethical dilemma for me; can I choose to do without, on behalf of the child? That's what I'm struggling with. On the other hand, when I'm looking there just aren't that many non-anonymous donors that appeal to me. That's the problem.
> –Mette (Teacher, in treatment with IUI-D)

At the core of this struggle lies a moral conflict between the perceived interests of the future child and a personal interest in both minimizing the involvement of the donor and making the optimal donor choice. The best match is also seen as one that provides the child with a positive (bio-genetic) foundation. Yet, as Mette expresses – along with other interviewees – it can be difficult to find a 'proper' identity release donor match, since the selection of donors is smaller for identity release donors.[2] In this regard the dilemma also pertain to looking after the best

---

[2]The supply of identity release donor sperm is smaller than for anonymous and non-anonymous donor sperm (donors with extended profiles). However, two of the world's largest sperm banks Cryos and European Sperm Bank – both based in Denmark – have experienced a major increase in donors who wish to be contactable donors (Oehlenschläger, 2015).

interest of the child in terms of either securing the best possible bio-genetic heritage from the male progenitor vs. securing a potential future social connection between the donor and the child that might support the child's sense of belonging and identity. In this way, it becomes a choice between the bio-genetic and social elements of relatedness.

Mette mainly views the donor in an instrumental fashion as providing the genetic material necessary for conception. The donor is also primarily perceived as non-kin, but she acknowledges that the genetic donation 'is culturally coded as meaningful and inscribed within systems of kinship' as described above, and that the donor is likely to be perceived as kin in the eyes of the child and by society at large. By drawing on her own biographical family experiences, she further substantiates the cultural expectations ascribed to the importance of genetic inheritance for kinship formation, and this adds to her dilemma of potentially side-stepping the best interest of the child in terms of donor disclosure. While this is at the core of the dilemma posed by many, others also emphasize the need to make sure that the child will actually be theirs even though the Non-identity release and identity release donor do not have any paternal rights over the child. Initially, Camilla considered using an anonymous donor to spare the child from false expectations regarding the potential presence of a biological father, but she decided that this was not her choice to make. As to her initial thoughts on choosing an Non-identity donor, she states:

> I think this choice [of selecting a Non-identity release donor] was more selfish actually, and that I kind of needed to be in control, yes… for it to be mine.
> –Camilla (Psychologist, pregnant through IUI-D)

The need to be able to claim an 'own child' as discussed in the previously chapter, provides a central argument for choosing a donor whose identity cannot be released at any point. Several of the women who have chosen a non-contactable donor explicitly state that they would not risk that the donor could make a claim on the child. Within the small group of women who chose an anonymous donor, some also explain that the process of handling an identity release donor was quite complex immediately after the new donor legislation was introduced, and that they were not comfortable with being in charge of handling/carrying the sperm, as was required at the time. For one of the interviewees, her choice of donor was primarily influenced by financial considerations. Identity release donor sperm is almost twice as expensive as anonymous sperm and she could not take the additional amount of money out of her monthly budget. Retrospectively, she explicitly states that she further justifies her choice by arguing that she does not want to give the child false expectations about the bio-genetic father. She also states that whatever donor option she chooses, the donor will not act as the father. She hopes that she and her family will be able to compensate for the loss and perhaps a potential partner will take on the role of the father. While most hope to meet a partner in the future, it seems reasonable to ask whether women who choose an anonymous donor are also more inclined to put their faith on the future presence of a social father? The rationales for choosing a certain donor do not seem to depend on such a wish. Only the interviewee who matched the donor criteria to those of a potential partner, emphasizes a strong wish for a social father to adopt her daughter. She also positions the donor in an instrumental manner as someone who primarily assists in the treatment phase.

Even though the donor is both represented as kin and/or as non-kin in the donor narratives, the donor is in general referred to as a donor and not as a father or biological father. Only one interviewee does refer to the donor as the father and another refers to him as a donor-father. It seems as if the terminology of the donor is used in an effort to demarcate clear kinship boundaries between the male progenitor and a potential social father. In this way, an effort is made to minimize the 'tension' inherent in the donor relationship along with any expectations of the future role of the identity release donor. Perhaps the evolving donor discourse involving an increased openness and augmented focus on donors makes their position in the kinship system even more difficult to transcend, and likewise the genetic connection more difficult to conceptualize. The women promote donor openness in the conception story that they plan to tell their children, but the kinship boundary work seems to protect them and their children from discursively constructing the donor as kin. Treating the donor as kin could create an amplified, idealized expectation that he will take part in the child's life at some point and form some kind of kin relation, whereas he is more likely above all to figure as symbolically present. The absence of a second social parent could increase such expectations, and if these expectations are not meet then the conception story could transform into one of deselection. As discussed in Chapter 4, the importance of the choice of solo motherhood being by design and not by chance functions as a safeguard for the child not feeling deselected by the biological father.

7.3.2 Donor Siblings

The choice of an identity release donor not only renders possible contact with the donor, but also allows for potential access to donor siblings. According to Danish legislation, a donor can help create 12 different families in Denmark. Within these families, there are no restrictions on the number of donor-siblings conceived by the donor's sperm (Ministry of Health, 2015). At the outset, children with the same donor are 'genetic strangers' (Hertz and Nelson, 2019, p. 4) or 'relative strangers' (Nordqvist and Smart, 2014, p. 9), linked together by shared genes but otherwise unknown to one another. By means of the donor number and the internet, many parents and donor-conceived children search for donor siblings and many connect, create new affiliations, networks, friendship and extended families (Andreassen, 2018, p. 12; Hertz and Nelson, 2019).

The interviewees who have already become solo mothers still have very young children and most are therefore not yet facing questions about the bio-genetic father. None of the women has yet made contact to other families with children from the same donor, one has registered with the donor number within a donor-sibling Facebook network whereas others have visited the network site but adopted a wait-and-see attitude. Overall, the women seem curious and forthcoming to the possibilities inherent in creating connections among potential donor siblings at some point in time. Due to the young age of their children, the possibilities however still seems premature and abstract. Based on the study data, it is not possible to predict whether the donor narratives will change as the children grow up. Previous research has shown that mothers tend to change their feelings about the donor after the child is born due to, among other factors, an increased awareness of certain characteristics observed to be dissimilar to the mothers (Zadeh et al., 2015, p. 6). In this regard, it seems likely that the categorization of the donor as kin vis-à-vis non-kin requires continuous management and negotiation and more flexible kin categorizations are likely to be considered necessary to account for and make sense of donor relations as their children grow up.

As with sperm donors, potential half-siblings created with the same donor sperm do not have a clear place in the kinship system either. Some of the women in this study see potential donor-siblings as a way for their children to create a network of children with similar conception stories. For other women, the existence of potential half-siblings is difficult to relate to, and despite a shared genetic connection amongst donor-siblings, the women find it difficult to categorize potential donor-siblings as kin.

> Saying that they are half-siblings makes my hair stand on end. Perhaps I can agree to saying that they are donor-siblings or say that they have the same genetic inheritance, but to me they are not half-siblings.
> –Maria (Teacher, pregnant with her second child through IVF)

The quotation from Maria illustrates how the meaning of bio-genetic links is negotiated and that in relation to potential donor siblings, the kinship boundary work proves challenging and illogical because it interferes with well-known ideas about kinship. As seen in the previous chapter, the women apply available kinship idioms in new ways to describe and renegotiate relatedness. In the same way do donor-conceived children – and their families – alter and invent existing kin terminology to reflect the new connections and affiliations created. For instance, some generally refer to donor siblings as 'diplings', 'halfies' or 'sperm siblings' or compare the new relations to those of well-known cousin relations, for instance (Hertz and Nelson, 2019, p. 219).

We also saw in the previous chapter that genetics are often either highlighted or downplayed depending on the type of relations formed and that the bio-genetic aspect played an essential part in the wish for an 'own' child and in the forming of solo mother families. In a similar way, it remains important for several women, including Maria, that their child can have a sibling (within their own solo mother family) conceived using the same donor. In this case, importance is attached to the shared bio-genetic link and seen to enhance the kin-relation among siblings. This supports a dynamic and relational understanding of identity and family formation and as pointed out by May: 'We must "do family" in order for a biological connection to mean something, and this meaning is not fixed in advance' (May, 2015, p. 487). Despite the importance attached to genetic inheritance as a foundation for creating kinship relations, a bio-genetic connection does not automatically translate into kin and family relations, as seen in the way the women in this study negotiate the position of both the sperm donor and potential donor-siblings.

Developments in medically assisted reproduction have paved the way for new kinship and family constellations and challenged more established conceptualizations of (bio-genetic) kinship. As seen in this chapter, negotiating the aspect of donor conception in particular seems to challenge well-known ideas about kinship since the donor's – and donor siblings' – place in the kinship system is not well established. Hence, clear kinship boundaries in relation to the donor are difficult to manage; sometimes the genetic donation is viewed merely as an instrumental means to an end, whilst at others, a personalized donation. The meaning attached to the donor changes, and even within the course of treatment, the donor is sometimes viewed as kin and sometimes as non-kin.

Chapter 8

Conclusion: Strategies for Life

In the beginning of this book, I took as my starting point a number of puzzling paradoxes that seem to characterize the developments and expansion of medically assisted reproduction. All these paradoxes revolve around the double feature of both imitating and destabilizing 'natural' forms of procreation and kinship relations. For instance, while being firmly based on biological processes and developed to 'give nature a helping hand' in establishing 'natural' kinship relations, they have increasingly been used to form 'new families' and have helped question biological versus social claims to kinship and family formation (Franklin, 2013a; McKinnon, 2015). General questions have been posed around to what extent this destabilization has helped challenge existing and endemic ideas and practises, and around what kinds of individual, social and legal responses they have provoked. It has been a salient issue in this book to explore their empirical manifestations within a Danish context and provide in-depth understandings of solo motherhood through assisted reproduction as a specific case to understand the lived realities and experiences of creating donor-conceived families.

In integrating the reciprocity between individuals, society and technology, this book seeks to understand and make visible the complex and multifaceted 'choreography between the natural and cultural' (Thompson, 2005, p. 177); between social and biogenetic aspects of kinship; between present realities and ideal conceptions and between personal and sociocultural narratives. The puzzling paradoxes discussed in the introduction appear to extend to the choice of embarking upon solo motherhood through donor insemination as well as resulting in questions particular to this choice. For instance, I asked, is the wish for a biological child of one's own greater due to the absence of the biogenetic father or are the social aspects of parenthood assessed to be more important when choosing to become the sole parent to a donor-conceived child? If a biological child of one's own is preferred, does that likewise imply that an identity-release donor is preferred in order for the child to be able to gain knowledge about its paternal biogenetic inheritance? These and many other questions and puzzles emerged as I moved through the research process, and it is evident from the empirical chapters that such questions often yield complex and at times ambiguous answers.

For instance, I find the choice to embark upon solo motherhood to be neither a first choice nor a second best. Identification is often a matter of 'complex (and often ambivalent) processes' (Brubaker and Cooper, 2000, p. 17). Contexts

Lived Realities of Solo Motherhood, Donor Conception
and Medically Assisted Reproduction, 177–186
Copyright © 2021 Tine Ravn
Published under exclusive licence by Emerald Publishing Limited
doi:10.1108/978-1-83909-115-520211010

change and biographical projects are revised on a continuous basis, potentially resulting in new expectations, perceptions and self-understandings. By addressing complex meaning-making processes through the narrative-biographical method, it is possible to track main narrative plot structures and transformative turning points that for instance signal a break between real and ideal, and identify how contradictions are negotiated and sometimes resolved through a number of different strategies and in dialogue with new opportunities and dependences.

Supported by the methodological and theoretical framework, this book details different forms of 'integrative processes' (Ginsburg, 1989, p. 135) related to pursuing solo motherhood through assisted reproduction. First of all, it analyses the decision-making process and the fertility treatment process through biographical and narrative plot structures and processes. This allows for insights into the complex rationalization, negotiation and adaptation processes which follow from the choice to have a child through donor conception. Through a focus on doing family and doing kinship, the book explores the lived experiences of relatedness as both an everyday and an imagined practice based on certain personal and culturally shaped ideals about doing family. When focusing on processes – however retrospectively – we see how self-understandings and life plans are both sustained and transformed as well as how participants seek to manage kinship boundaries in terms of the 'conflicting significance of nature versus nurture' (Nordqvist and Smart, 2014, p. 150) and how these boundary shifts are being drawn in new and sometimes unexpected ways. A central finding in this study comprises the complex and shifting boundary work with regard to donor relations, and with regard to 'natural' processes, in which the latter for instance relates to how new lines for fertility treatment procedures are often pushed in the process towards motherhood.

Process in this book is not only to be understood as a matter of becoming, negotiating and doing, emphasizing discursive phenomena; rather, as shown throughout the book, it is equally a matter of navigating within established and normatively regulated practices and structures that appear as 'given' and which both limit and enable courses of action. Social changes related to legislative rights and benefits, changed socio-demographic compositions and greater variance in family structures have helped expand the possibilities for identification but at the same time, objectified and naturalized societal expectations also continue to provide grounds for legitimating the decision to go it alone.

8.1 Solo Motherhood: Contextual Particularities and Life Trajectories

In the introduction, I argued that Denmark provides an interesting context for studying solo motherhood in relation to medically assisted reproduction due to its status as a welfare society with permissive MAR legislation and free access to fertility treatment within the public health care system. Moreover, the Danish position as 'the fertility hub of Scandinavia' (Kroløkke et al., 2019, p. 1) and its hosting of the world's largest sperm bank, Cryos International, carry with it exoteric implications extending well beyond its national context. Hence, despite certain national particularities, the Danish case is firmly anchored in the greater technological and sociocultural transformations described and analysed in this book.

As to the particular political and discursive environment of the governing of this field in the Danish setting, the analysis overall points to a change towards more inclusive family understandings and an increased normalization of reproductive technologies. The women in this research consider the production of equal rights to fertility treatment, as granted in 2007, to be the most important social change underlying their decision to embark upon solo motherhood and this supports the more general observation that rights and benefits are decisive when 'claiming family' and imperative for cultural acceptance and recognition (May, 2015, p. 483). The change in legislative practises and the concomitant medical and financial resources provided support the realization of solo mother families and are seen as a public signal of acceptance in underlining this particular route to motherhood and family formation as legitimate and acceptable. While the policy analysis in this book merely reflects a change in policy position due, among other factors, to social and technological trans-formations and discursive changes, the women's narratives in turn, illustrate the reciprocity between discourse and legislation in influencing normalization pro-cesses. The changes in legislation have helped transform institutionalized and 'established-ways-of-doing-things' (Jenkins, 2008, p. 40) and influenced the women's biographies not only by specifically expanding 'the field of possibilities' (Foucault, 1983, p. 221) in making it a less stratified choice, but also by making it a more acceptable one.

In general, the increased pluralization of family constellations as well as their growing societal acceptance adds to the normalization of the women's choice to embark upon solo motherhood, and comprises a decisive factor in motivating and justifying their decision. It broadens the possibility of identifying with other single parents and/or blended families and most importantly, the women believe that their children will be able to identify with many of their peers who also have experiences of family constellations which differ from the nuclear family model.

As I interviewed the women in this study, I collected more and more life story narratives that revealed diversity rather than homogeneity, and the complexity regarding biographical particularities, experiences, motivations and so forth were notable. Furthermore, while they confirmed existing knowledge about solo mothers being professional and financially secure women, they diverged in terms of age, geographical location, type and length of education, and civil status (previous marriages, existing children etc.). The many biographical narratives, quotations and excerpts presented throughout the book clearly illustrate indi-vidual complexity, but also provide pieces that combine to create a collective portrait.

When comparing the lived experiences as expressed through the plot story of the women's biographical narratives, shared themes, motivations and common plots could be traced. In general, the theme of *independence and nurture* inter-weaves sequences of biographical experiences with understandings of self. Com-mon plot structures related to education, employment, periods spent abroad and relocations among others, reflect a high degree of independent decision-making. Furthermore, choice of occupation often intersects with elements of nurture, and internal and external self-identifications of being great with children and taking on the role of nurturers are highlighted as both significant biographical and narrative elements. On the whole, the position of motherhood remains a strong identifier throughout the women's narratives and seems impossible to transcend. It is projected into future visions of motherhood, and self-understandings and life plans are transformed accordingly.

The transitional marker of not having found the right partner is a common plot in the life stories and shared turning points often include the ending of short or long-term relationships and increasing concerns about fertility decline. Moreover, experiencing a limited prospect of finding a partner initiates a process of reworking their initial family ideals and negotiating a departure from them. The women in this study would all have preferred to have a child within a relationship. A key message in the interviews has been that the decision to embark upon solo motherhood is about the active and positive choice to have a child and not the active choice not to have a partner. In the decision-making process, two types of resources are emphasized as profound in contemplating solo motherhood: (a) the ability to be a qualified parent in order to be able to secure the psychological wellbeing of the child. Abilities such as 'responsibility' and 'emotional maturity' are stressed as important, and (b) to secure a safe and stable environment by securing a permanent job and providing a suitable home and social network. The type of resources highlighted and the limited prospect of finding a partner and increasing concerns about age and fertility decline as key motivating factors are in keeping with other studies within this field (see Bock, 2000; Frederiksen et al., 2011; Golombok, 2015; Graham, 2013; Murray and Golombok, 2005a).

The choice to embark upon solo motherhood constitutes a moral decision and a moral dilemma, primarily due to the fact that their children will grow up without the presence and/or knowledge of their biological fathers. This dilemma regarding the 'need for a father' (Gamble, 2009) causes much ambivalence and contemplation. The women justify their choice in several ways; for instance they believe they will be able to provide their children with happy childhoods where they will be surrounded by close and loving relations and that it will not be detrimental for their children to grow up without a father. They substantiate this by the child's positive conception story and early-disclosure of being donor-conceived. Some also refer to existing research showing that children generally thrive very well in solo mother families. In addition, all hope and some plan more actively for a future partner who will be able to act as a social father/second partner for their child. While the contemplations above are in line with existing research within the area of solo motherhood (see Chapter 1), the polysemy and ambivalence of the concept of 'choice' are less framed as a matter of 'constraint' (Graham, 2014) in the women's narratives and I analyse this as a transformation of real and ideal sense-making in the process towards motherhood. The designation of a *'narrative of best choice'* aims to capture the paradoxical features of the choice to contemplate solo motherhood as being neither their initial choice nor a second best. It is a choice by design and not by chance and about choosing a child, not deselecting a partner. Moreover, the 'best choice narrative' refers to the strategic shaping of chosen life plans in relation to life chance possibilities and limitations. It is also a narrative about strategies – in the told story as well as in the lived life – to minimize the ambivalence and uncertainties that not only ensue from the edict to individually manage 'the reflexively organized trajectory of the self' (Giddens, 1991, p. 85), but also that follow from embarking upon a less 'standardized' route to family formation.

The shared characteristics and motivations found in this study both add to and partly confirm existing knowledge within the field of solo motherhood. While this book does not include a comparative study as such, it seems that the women in this study are relatively younger compared to international studies at where women embarking upon solo motherhood are often reported to be in their late thirties and early forties (Bock, 2000; Grill, 2005; Golombok, 2015, 2020; Graham, 2013; Jadva et al., 2009a; Malmquist et al., 2019; Mannis, 1999). More than a third of the women in this research initiated treatment in their early thirties. The wish to become a young mother, to potentially have more than one child and an awareness about actual or potential age-related fertility issues constitute main motivational factors for starting treatment at what is considered to be a young age in the medical system. However, when coupled with experiences of not having found the right partner, many experience the shared feeling of being pressed for time. Paradoxically, it seems as if the younger group of women to a greater extent face contradictory societal expectations; on the one hand, they are very much aware of the national and medical awareness campaigning around fertility reduction factors such as age and the advantages of having children earlier, and on the other hand they seem – to a greater extent – to challenge the expectations inherent in the structure and content related to the 'normal biography'.

8.2 Medically Assisted Reproduction: Redefining the Meaning of Kinship and Family

At its core, the book is engaged with how biogenetic and social connections (nature-culture) are defined and given meaning when family and kinship relations are literally and actively created by the women in this study. This has been explored through the women's strategies for creating life through assisted reproduction and building life as a solo mother, for instance in terms of the strategies used to motivate the decision to parent alone and the strategies invoked to claim an own child through the use of donor conception. The book seeks to provide new understandings of how single women 'do' family, identity and kinship and how the choice to create life as a solo mother is continuously rationalized and normalized. While the decision – and the child's conception – is for life, the book shows that the considerations and understandings of what is 'given' and what is 'made' in terms of establishing kinship and family relations (Carsten, 2004, p. 9), are dynamic and variant and help to shape familial narratives of e.g. mother-child relations and donor/donor sibling relations in a way at where perceptions and practices are both reproduced and innovated at once.

In this regard, the case of solo motherhood is explored in its own right; in an intrinsic fashion with a view to the distinctiveness particularly pertaining to embarking upon solo motherhood through assisted reproduction. For instance, the book provides a first account of going through fertility treatment as a single woman and through these personal narratives, shows how boundaries of 'natural processes' are redefined. The decision-making process and the importance attached to biological and social aspect of kinship point to the above-mentioned theme of both sustaining and re-defining perceptions of 'natural processes' in terms of family formation, motherhood and procreation. Processes of naturalization and normalization interlink with changed contexts and circumstances and consequently with biographical revisions taking place. The process of undergoing fertility treatment is highly interrelated with such processes and shaped by the relationship between sociocultural discourse and biological materiality and the techno-scientific intervention of reproductive technology.

From a general point of view, the women in this study adopt a positive attitude towards reproductive technologies. They emphasize the expansion of their reproductive choices and see them as supporting a morally responsible route to solo motherhood. They are conceived of as a 'hope technology' (Franklin, 1997, p. 192) and the women put their faith in them in terms of assisting them with fulfilling their wish to have a child on their own. However, the process of undergoing fertility treatment yield more ambiguous experiences and in keeping with other studies of patients undergoing treatment (particularly IVF), their treatment processes can be viewed as an 'emotional roller-coaster' (Thompson, 2005, p. 93); as becoming a 'way of life' (Franklin, 1997, p. 131) and reproductive technology as a 'catalyst for disruption' (Becker, 2000, p. 266) in terms of its emotional and physical impacts.

Several women explicitly apply the 'roller-coaster' metaphor or describe a process of experiencing 'ups and downs' to account for the emotional strain of undergoing treatment. The alternating states between hope and discouragement relates to the emotional stress of 'not knowing' whether treatment will result in pregnancy and motherhood, and I find this to cause the greatest strain and vulnerability. The emotional and physical strains of treatment do however reinforce each other and throughout the treatment process, the bodily processes comprise the primary focus in the medical procedures. Part of the strain related to the 'unknown' also includes insecurities related to how the body is going to perform in the process. The 'unmanageable' aspect of how bodies will react to the treatment procedures speaks to the 'agency of bodily matter' (Haraway, 2004a; Lykke, 2010) and to the interdependence of both techno-cultural discourse and biological materiality in the process (Haraway, 2004a, p. 67). At the same time, efforts are made to manage bodies through techno-cultural discourses, and through individual measures performed as well. As to the latter, 'biological responsibility' (Rose, 2001, p. 19) is enacted in a number of ways, among others in regard to life style changes, adhering to the time-tabled nature of treatment and to the participation in treatment decisions, for instance in regard to the number of embryos to be transferred.

Furthermore, in detailing how the women in this study conceive of and engage in assisted reproduction, I show how the interplay of technological objectification and individual agency inherent in the 'ontological choreography' (Thompson, 2005) is performed and how the women seem to adopt a more instrumental approach as treatment progresses and they become more familiar with treatment procedures. In this regard, boundaries are moved in the process and understandings of 'natural' processes are to some extent reworked. There is a tendency to want to begin treatment that comes as close to 'natural' processes of procreation as possible for a number of reasons. If the form of treatment they are undergoing proves unsuccessful, there is a similar tendency to wanting to move on to a next phase of treatment as a response to changed conditions and contexts.

With regard to the aspects of biogenetic and social relatedness, these are weighted differently in the women's family and kinship perceptions and practices depending on the type of relation, i.e. relation to the child, the donor or broader family and network relations. For instance, when embarking upon solo motherhood through donor conception, the desire for an 'own child' brings with it a number of considerations that relate to the importance ascribed to both biogenetic and social aspects. This is a complex matter with no clear or consistent boundaries drawn. For instance, sometimes genetics is merely about passing on certain physical traits whereas sometimes it is taken to be highly intertwined with biological and social processes of attachment and identification. The evidence suggest that the meanings attached to biogenetic and social aspects of relatedness are shaped by individual particularities (e.g. upbringing, line of employment etc.), by the fertility treatment process itself and by prevailing cultural narratives on procreation and family formation. Based on these findings and the concept of 'strategic naturalizing' (Thompson, 2005, p. 274), I point to five main strategies used in this process that details how the women (1) interlink biology, motherhood and attachment/nurture; (2) how they naturalize the interlinkage of motherhood and womanhood, (3) and relate maternity to biogenetic ties and paternity to social ties. Furthermore, the women are found to (4) highlight the importance of mother-child resemblance as a basis for identity and belonging and (5) safeguard the mother-child relation through the biogenetic link in order to secure and argue for an 'own child'.

While the biogenetic link remains a very important aspect in the desire for a child of one's own, the distinction between biological and social relations becomes much more fluid when the women in this study create close networks of family, friends and acquaintances around themselves and their (future) children. Supporting networks are mobilized and it is evident from the biographical narratives that children born into solo mother families are also born into an extended family and broader social network consisting of various kinds of social relations such as the women's parents and siblings, close male and female friends, extended family relations that are reinforced, arrangements that are established with substitute grandparents, as well as involvement in physical and virtual networks with other (solo) mothers. Many women tell of friends and relatives that are brought closer; sometimes friends are made into kin and designated as such, and in several cases they are considered to be closer than biological relatives. By using well-known idioms for kinship to refer to non-biogenetic relations, the women both draw on existing 'kinship thinking' while also extending the meaning of relatedness beyond biological ties.

When the interviewees define the concept of family and construct new meaningful family narratives, the nuclear family as 'the family we live by' is challenged and re-negotiated to better reflect 'the families we live with' (Gillis, 1996, p. xv). The women's own experiences with specific family constellations and previous relationships enter into their perceptions of what constitutes a family but I find that the increased possibilities to construct new narratives of 'doing family' which depart from the nuclear family model, extend beyond their own family experiences and reflect more general societal changes in family demographics.

When conceptualizing and relating to the donor, the duality of biological and social connections take on yet another meaning in the women's narratives. As established by existing research, the genetic donation poses a paradoxical tension: while the donation itself is embedded within existing kinship systems, donors will often not take an active part in the child's upbringing, but will remain as merely 'imagined fathers' (Hertz, 2002, p. 1), and a kind of 'absence presence' (Zadeh et al., 2015, p. 3; Nordqvist and Smart, 2014, p. 107) at least until the child reaches adulthood. In the wake of the importance of genetic inheritance and greater donor openness being established through cross-country policy measures, comes the question of whether donors are conceptualized as kin or as non-kin? The distinct Danish two-way donor model of allowing for both donors and recipients to decide the degree of openness surrounding the donation (i.e. anonymous, open and known donation) further allows for a comparison between the different rationales given by the interviewees as to why different donor programmes are chosen.

In general, the choice of choosing the 'right' donor is made after careful considerations about respective donor types and their implications for the child in regard to the paternal inheritance. The choice of donor often constitutes a moral dilemma with regards to the best interest of the child, at the heart of which lies the question whether the women ought to deny their child the opportunity to form a relation to its paternal inheritance, even though the donor will not be a father and may not desire any prolonged contact with the child. The main rationale for choosing an identity-release donor is to give the child the opportunity to learn more about, and meet, the donor, and the attitude that this should be the child's decision instead of the mother's. Still, many of the women are concerned that this opportunity could create false hope and cause the donor to take on too much significance for the child. Several arguments are framed for choosing a donor that cannot be contacted and the concern about false hope constitutes one of them. The women who have chosen an identity-release donor hope that the donor narratives created between mother and child will help mitigate possible let-downs. It is evident that clear kinship boundaries in donor relations are difficult to manage; even within the fertility treatment process, the donor can for instance be regarded as both kin and non-kin. The manner in which the women position both the donor and potential donor-siblings underlines that biogenetic connections do not automatically translate into kin but that 'we must "do family" in order for a biological connection to mean something' (May, 2015, p. 487).

8.3 Concluding Reflections: The Question of (Im)mutability

> The history one is born into is always so naturalised until you
> reflect back on it and then suddenly everything is meaningful – the
> multiple layers of insertion in a landscape of social and cultural
> histories all of a sudden pops out.
>
> – (Haraway, 2000, pp. 5–6)

If I am to sum up the current book in one sentence, 'strategies for life' seems to capture its essential elements; the book explores solo motherhood through assisted reproduction as a particular route to experiencing motherhood, and explores how life plans, strategies and biographical revisions are transformed in the tension between the individual and the social, and between nature and culture. In this way, it thematizes some of the core elements for and in life: procreation, identity and relatedness.

The women's narratives highlight individual experiences, and the close navigation to more endemic perspectives on 'naturalized' kinship thinking, for instance in relation to motivating and legitimating the decision to have a child of ones' own, partly reflects challenges and issues particular to this pathway to motherhood. Hence, a biological foundation remains important, an observation which seems to be reinforced by the fact that the women will be the sole social parent who is also genetically connected to the child. While solo motherhood has been explored as a case in its own right, it can also be construed as a case that mirrors greater processes and implications of change in the interrelationship between reproductive technologies and sociocultural processes, showing how existing ideas and practices of family and kinship are both being reproduced and challenged in the wake of new possibilities and rights provided. Biographies illuminate the relations between individual life stories and societal processes and uncover how structural changes influence individual life trajectories. In this regard, individual narratives 'embodies – and gives us insight into – what is possible and intelligible within a specific social context' (Chase, 2005, p. 667). The ambiguity at play when incorporating the significance of genes into existing thinking about kinship and family formation, are found in several other studies exploring 'new' kinship making in relation to reproductive technologies (for instance Nordqvist and Smart, 2014; Carsten, 2004; Thompson, 2005), with these studies supporting the view of social innovation in this area of kinship as 'an actively negotiated process of continuous, and often strategic recomposition out of varied elements' which both reproduce and modify established kinship thinking (Franklin, 2013b, p. 4).

While these more general observations point to a shared discursive space for action in which new elements can be combined and practised, it is exactly the individual studies which more clearly mark out the intelligible limits of kinship thinking and which empirical findings delineate how particular elements are combined. Caught between visions of familiar ideals and the want of a child of one's own, the women in this study are perhaps not bordering the discursive limits available, but their ways of thinking and practising kinship add to the normalization of 'new family' constellations and help answer the question of when and why more 'naturalized' kinship categories are either reproduced or reconfigured. Hence, the women's narratives reflect a continuing negotiation of normalization and naturalization processes as to ways of 'doing' family and kinship within existing sociocultural structures.

Exploring the lived realities of embarking upon solo motherhood through the particular lens of the biographical-narrative method also allows for more holistic understandings into retrospective processes of ascribing meaning to past experiences and choices. The construction of meaningful narratives, however, does not preclude the complexities, ambiguities and continuous negotiations that follow from recrafting biographical projects. This study has empirically explored both new and more familiar transformations and interlinkages between individual actions, societal structures and technological innovations from the a priori assertion that they take on meaning and definition through each other. In this regard, the purpose has been to explore these interlinkages and 'multiple layers' to explore how cultural particularities – such as equality in access to reproduction, public available treatment, welfare structures, the distinct Danish donor programme, particular cultural discourses of family formation, motherhood and so forth – have influenced the women's decision to embark upon solo motherhood and form 'new families'. Still, more national and cross-country research concerning the lived experiences of solo motherhood through donor conception could well be expanded upon in the future so as to further substantiate and nuance the findings in this book. Overall, with the increasing accessibility of medically assisted reproduction (e.g. double/embryo donation); advances in reproductive technologies (e.g. egg-freezing and mitochondrial donation) and increased possibilities to learn about, connect with and build new network relations with donor siblings through DNA databases, donor sibling registries and social media, new questions keep emerging as to the meaning of relatedness and the duality of nature and nurture. Additional research could further our understandings of new and shifting ways of forming families and provide more answers to the many – often normative – questions raised. Despite applying the category of solo mothers throughout this study, I hope to have shown that to understand the complexity of lived realities demand as much focus on diversity as on commonalities and that family can be 'done' in many ways.

Appendix 1: Conducting the Study: Research Design and Methodology

A.1 Research Design

The research study, on which this book is based, apply a multi-level and multi-method approach. It is situated within an explorative, interpretative and qualitative design and its scientific theoretical approach draws on the concept of 'situated knowledge' (Haraway, 1988), embodying a duality between subjectivity (constructivism) and objectivity (realism). The book revolves around an empirically based investigation of solo motherhood through donor insemination, with a view to explore the experience, meaning and use of assisted reproduction and its influence on reproductive practices and processes of normalization, identity construction and family and kinship formation. To this end, the study makes use of the narrative biographical method as its primary method of inquiry alongside expert interviews, field observations and policy analysis. Personal narratives of the lived experiences of solo motherhood, kinship and assisted reproduction are analysed, and the ways in which wider sociocultural narratives are adopted, resisted and transformed – for instance discursive, technological, personal and legislative possibilities and constraints within particular sociocultural contexts – are explored.

A.1.1 Biographical Narrative Interview Study

The study comprises 22 biographical narrative interviews with single women or solo mothers, and at the time of interview, the women differed as to whether they were in fertility treatment, had become pregnant or had conceived a child through insemination (IUI-D) or IVF (see Table A1).The biographical narrative interviews were conducted during the period of September 2014 to March 2015.

The biographical narrative method and the use of in-depth interviews are well suited to address the interlinking of personal and sociocultural narratives. To this end, biographies not only reflect the particularities of individual lives, trajectories, choices, experiences and events but also the shared social, structural and cultural contexts which enable and constrain individual stories and actions (Corbally and O'Neill, 2014; Chamberlayne et al., 2000; Hoerning, 1996; Roberts, 2002). Biographies are themselves social constructions and constituted by social

Lived Realities of Solo Motherhood, Donor Conception
and Medically Assisted Reproduction, 187–198
Copyright © 2021 Tine Ravn
Published under exclusive licence by Emerald Publishing Limited
doi:10.1108/978-1-83909-115-520211011

Table A1. Division of Participants in Terms of Fertility Treatment.

Dimensions	In Fertility Treatment	Pregnancy Achieved	Given Birth	Total
IUH-D	2	5	4	11
IVF (ICSI)	6 (incl. 1 + ICSI)	1	4 (incl. 2 + ICSI)	11
Total	8	6	8	22

processes, since both the lived life (the experienced life history, biographical facts) and the told story (the self-narrated story, text) reflect social interaction involving both a micro, mesa and macro level (Antoft and Thomsen, 2005; Järvinen, 2005). Analytically, the method allows for a bridging of the dynamic and dialectic relation between micro-macro levels (agency-structure).

The biographical narrative method is also applied in this study due to its strengths in eliciting sensitive personal accounts and providing nuanced under-standings of complex meaning-making processes (e.g. decision-making, course of fertility treatment, normalization strategies, rationalization of biological and social aspect of kinship). The method is also suitable for reaching in-depth and holistic understandings through broader life stories/transformative experiences and for studying 'lived realities' and narratively explore life plans vs. life changes as well as breaks between real and ideal.

The time dimensions of past, present and future constitute a substantial element within the interpretation of personal accounts (Roberts, 2002). Individuals' pasts, family generations and institutions, among others, influence the individual shaping of life histories. Within these, central events, transitions and milestones represent significant life story aspects, experienced and interpreted by each individual in a sequence of events, where one event, not unexpectedly, follows earlier life events. Nonetheless, these are also interpretatively structured by individuals according to a beginning, a middle and an ending which provide them with a narrative nature. Considerable events may be characterized as turning points at which the individual management of these situations in particular, will impact on the future life course (Hoerning, 2001; Antoft and Thomsen, 2005; Heinz and Krüger, 2001). The concepts of life-planning as opposed to life chances (Thomsen, 2005) provide relevant analytical notions within the conceptual framework of biographical research. Life courses are to varying degrees 'characterized by discontinuities and shifting patterns of life-planning'. Life-plans, furthermore, depend on the life chances available (structures of possibilities and limitations), which again, depend on historical circumstances, social institutions such as family, education, social policy and economy, as well as on social characteristics attached to gender, class, ethnicity etc. (Heinz and Krüger, 2001).

In general, in this book, I wish to explore the interaction between personal narratives of solo mothers including their experiences, interpretations and meaning constructions and how sociocultural and technological changes and developments come across as significant in their life stories.

A.2 Data Collection: Sample and Recruitment

A.2.1 Sample

The table below display the division of participants at the time of the interview according to the dimensions of whether the women are undergoing fertility treatment ($n = 8$); have become pregnant ($n = 6$) or have conceived a child ($n = 8$). The table furthermore accounts for the most recent type of treatment procedure applied (if both insemination and IVF (and ICSI) have been applied, the participant will figure under the latter). The sample includes variation with regard to the *processual* character of applying medically assisted reproduction and the different past and present fertility treatment experiences enables a diverse set of processual experiences and a comparative perspective to their biographical work and to the presence of different life course turning points.

The interviewees are located across Denmark, although with a concentration of informants in and close to the two largest cities Copenhagen and Aarhus. Two of the Danish participants live abroad; one participant is based in Scandinavia and has participated in fertility treatment in Denmark, whereas the participant located in Belgium underwent treatment there. One participant is German and lives in Germany but for several years, she has participated in fertility treatments at a private clinic in Copenhagen. At the time of interview, the women were aged between 29 and 40 with the average age being 36.4. The majority of participants have completed medium-cycle higher educations, while the remaining have completed long cycle higher educations. The women in the sample represent a variety of professional backgrounds (see Table A2).

A.2.2 Recruitment and Sample Strategy

In the collection of biographical narrative interviews, a multiple and purposeful sampling strategy was employed. The invitation/information letter to participate in the study was disseminated through different channels. Five public fertility clinics representing all regions of Denmark agreed to disseminate information about the study. The invitation was also disseminated through two national online resources for single mothers by choice; an open Facebook group created and administered by Signe Fjord, a well-known author, solo mother and speaker within the field, as well as a closed online forum for single mothers by choice. As additional sampling strategies, a few interviewees were recruited through a network of acquaintances (for instance the friend of a colleague's cousin) and one interviewee was recruited through snow ball sampling and thus from among the acquaintances of an existing interviewee. The different sampling approaches were applied in order to access the field in general and reach a broader and more diverse group of solo mothers to facilitate an 'information oriented' selection of informants (Bo, 2005, p. 71). For this reason, the recruitment process was also specified and intensified during data

Table A2. Overview of Interview Participants: Demographic Data.

Interviewee	Age	Nationality	Residence	Education	Profession	Previous Marriage/No. of Children	Fertility Treatment/ Donor Type	Public and/or Private Clinic
1. Mette (pseudonym)	39	Danish	Northern Jutland	Teacher	Adult education	–	In treatment (IUI-D), identity-release donor	Public
2. Kira Poulsen	35	Danish	Copenhagen	Archaeologist and pedagogue	Nursery teacher	–	Pregnant with twins (IUI-D), anonymous donor	Private
3. Charlotte (pseudonym)	38	Danish	Aarhus	Physiotherapy	Physiotherapist	–	In treatment (IUI-D), identity-release donor	Public
4. Camilla (pseudonym)	30	Danish	Aarhus	Psychology	Psychologist	Daughter from previous marriage	Pregnant (IUI-D), identity-release donor	Private
5. Tanja Lønnqvist	37	Danish	Aarhus	Export engineering	Export engineer	–	Daughter, 2 months old, (IUI-D), anonymous donor	Public
6. Henriette Thomsen	39	Danish	Silkeborg	Physiotherapy	Physiotherapist	–	Pregnant (IUI-D), anonymous donor	Public
7. Christina Hansen	32	Danish	Herning	Social work	Social worker	–	In treatment (IVF), anonymous donor	Public
8. Tina Albertsen	37	Danish	Herning	Retail management	Management position in retail	–	Daughter, 6 months old (IUI-D), anonymous donor	Private

	Age	Nationality	City	Education	Occupation		Treatment/Child	Public/Private
9. Ditte (pseudonym)	43	Danish	Belgium	Law degree	Lawyer	–	Daughter, 1 year old (IUI-D, IVF, ICSI), identity-release donor	Public (no reimbursement)
10. Marie Louise (pseudonym)	29	Danish	Aarhus	Nursing education + psychology	Lecturer	–	Pregnant (IUI-D), identity-release donor	Public
11. Emma (pseudonym)	31	Danish	Odense	Nursing education	Nurse	–	Pregnant (IUI-D), identity-release donor (+anonymous donor)	Public + private
12. Anne Reimar	39	Danish	Copenhagen	Pharmaconomist	Pharmaconomist	Divorced	In treatment (IVF), anonymous donor (henceforward identity-release donor)	Public
13. Cecilie (pseudonym)	36	Danish	Copenhagen	Nursing education	Nurse	–	Son, 3 months old (IVF), identity-release donor	Public
14. Maria Laustsen	35	Danish	Silkeborg	Teacher	Teacher	Donor-conceived child (IVF)	Pregnant (IVF), donor with extended profile (non-contactable)	Private

Table A2. *(Continued)*

Interviewee	Age	Nationality	Residence	Education	Profession	Previous Marriage/No. of Children	Fertility Treatment/ Donor Type	Public and/or Private Clinic
15. Thilde Petersen	33	Danish	Aarhus	Nursing education	Nurse	–	Son, 3 months old (IUI-D, IVF, ICSI), donor with extended profile (non-contactable)	Public and private
16. Mille Tikjøb	39	Danish	Aarhus	Animal assistant	Insurance consultant	–	Daughter, 2 years old (IUI-D), identity-release donor	Private
17. Sarah (pseudonym)	32	Danish	Smaller city north of Copenhagen	Pedagogue	Pedagogue	Donor-conceived child (IUI-D)	Pregnant (IUI-D), identity-release donor	Private
18. Karoline Larsen	40	Danish	Copenhagen	The Royal Danish Academy of Fine Arts	Artist	–	In treatment (IUI-D, IVF), identity-release donor	Public
19. Anna (pseudonym)	40	Danish	Scandinavia	PhD	Associate Professor	Daughter from previous marriage	In treatment (IUI-D, IVF), identity-release donor (+anonymous donor, undecided about future donor)	Private

20. Karen Marie Dahl	40	Norwegian	Copenhagen	Pedagogue	Support worker	Widow	Pregnant (IVF), identity-release donor	Public and private
21. Elizabeth (pseudonym)	40	Danish	Copenhagen	Office administration training	Insurance company	—	In treatment (IVF), identity-release donor	Private and public
22. Esther D.	37	German	Germany	Teacher and Pedagogue	Nursery teacher	—	In treatment (IUH-D, IVF, ICSI), identity-release donor	Private

collection. The interviewees recruited initially only comprised single women with experience of insemination with donor semen and not IVF with donor semen. In order to include the latter group, the invitation to participate was changed during data collection, and I expanded the dissemination strategy to include three private fertility clinics in order to address this group in particular.

All but two interviews were arranged through email correspondence, and all interviewees received written information about the objectives of the research project, the option to be anonymous and the type of interview in which they would potentially participate. The potential participants received this background information in the initial planning of the interviews in order for them to finally accept or decline the initial invitation to participate. All but one interview took place face-to-face. The majority of interviews were carried out in the interviewees' homes whilst a few interviewees preferred to meet at a café of their choice. The interview with the German participant was conducted via Skype for logistical reasons.

A2.3 Collecting Data: Interview Design

For the interview design, the procedure for biographical narrative interviews as outlined by Rosenthal (1993, 2004) and introduced by Fritz Schütze in the 1970s was applied. The method implies a rather stringent temporal procedure with the aim of encouraging 'extempore narration' of experiences (Rosenthal, 1993, p. 1) rather than to elicit arguments and theoretical accounts alike. In this regard, interviewer intervention is minimized (Wengraf, 2001, p. 112). As stated in Corbally and O'Neill (2014, p. 36), the attempt to uncover

> ...what participants want to say, not what the researcher wants them to say (...) is useful in ascertaining how people make sense of themselves in their life stories and enables the researcher to study how participants account for their life experiences.

The interviewer opens the interview by posing an open question requesting that the interviewees/biographers tell their life story or part of it (Rosenthal, 2004, p. 50). This main narration is not interrupted with questions by the interviewer, who only takes notes and encourages further narration by paralinguistic expressions or small prompts. In this first part, I asked the interviewees to tell their life story starting from when they finished lower secondary school. By starting at this point in time, I wished to take account of stories from the formative years of adolescence, including educational choices up until the present day. Interestingly, several women included specific childhood experiences which they considered to be of great importance for the story told.

In the next phase of interviewing, internal narrative questions are posed in which questioning relates to and elaborates on the issues already mentioned. Questions and issues of particular interest to the researcher, the external narrative questions, are therefore not asked until the last phase of the interview (Rosenthal, 2004, p. 50). Although there is disagreement around whether a specific narrative interview exists (Andrews, 2012), the interviewer aims to elicit narrative telling and minimize the use of 'why questions'. Furthermore, contradictions are not highlighted, and rather than 'testing' your interpretations in the interview, you ask them to elaborate on a given issue. Similarly, you focus on being an active listener rather than interfering with questions (Phoenix, 2013).

The main themes explored in the interview guide relate to the decision-making process (ranging from micro-macro influences); the process of fertility treatment; social relations and family formation, and future plans. As part of each interview, I asked the women to draw a relational map and through a number of concentric circles, write down the closest and most important people in their life. The proximity to the inner circle then reflects the closeness of the relationships. The approach of employing relational maps is inspired by Roseneil's (2006) psycho-social study of intimacy and sociability. The main objective of including this technique in the interview design was to explore the women's social networks and the construction of relatedness in order to further explore in what way the interplay of biogenetic and social ties influence family and kinship conceptions and actual family constructions. The map functioned as a concrete tool to facilitate talk about the often complex character of social networks and family constellations. I found the drawing of maps to be highly efficient not only for opening up descriptions of various network constellations, but also as a technique to elicit narrative telling about their families and friends, among others. The relational maps and the stories they elicit also formed the basis for a subsequent set of related questions of mere abstract and existential character. The interviews were recorded and transcribed verbatim and subsequently coded through a thematically oriented and explorative coding strategy in the software programme NVivo, which is designed to facilitate the management and analysis of empirical material. The analytical strategy was constructed as an iterative process whose elements of a thematical cross-case comparison, within-case analysis (of biographical profiles and the narrative content/structure) and an analysis of contrasting plot structures constantly informed and reinforced one another.

A.3 Ethical Considerations

Adhering to ethical guidelines and professional standards of research integrity remains imperative in any kind of research, not least in biographical research in which narrating one's life history often implies conveying personal and sensitive information. A number of elements pertaining to responsible research practices are important to consider throughout the entire research process as matters of research ethics as 'ethics in practice' (Fujii, 2012, p. 717) is an ongoing concern related to the entire research process.

A.3.1 Transparency and Informed Consent

Securing transparency relates to providing clear information about the research objectives. Such information was given prior to and after the interview to secure that the women's consent to participate in the study was given on an informed basis (see above). In the background material as well as in the beginning of each interview, it was also emphasized that it was entirely up to each participant to decide how much information to share with me. The possibility to see transcriptions/quotations beforehand also aims to increase transparency in terms of how interview contributions were to be reported.

A.3.2 Confidentiality and Anonymity

Due to the very personal and potentially sensitive character of sharing one's life story, all interviewees were given the option of anonymity. It was evident from the beginning of data collection that it was important for some participants to disseminate their stories in a non-anonymous fashion to stand by their choice and tell their story. Several models of representation were then applied according to the preferred choice of each participant. Some choose to be anonymous in which revealing details are not included, whereas others chose to use only their first name but with their full stories (see Table A2). Others again have chosen to appear with a pseudonym but with demographic details included. A few interviewees wished to read the transcripts before making a final decision regarding anonymity. A small number of interviewees also wished to receive the final transcription as a form of documentation similar to that of diary recordings. As this book is based on the PhD thesis 'Strategies for Life: Lived Realities of Solo Motherhood, Kinship and Medically Assisted Reproduction', all participants were contacted in connection with the making of this book to give consent to their interviews being included in the book, too. Participants were also asked to assess the level of information the wished to provide. The majority choose to continue with the model originally chosen.

A.3.3 Analytical Presentation/Reporting of Findings

The reporting of individual life histories not only relate to transparency but also to the issue of avoiding misrepresentations in the analysis. Following up with clarifying questions, a review of unclear transcription passages and a thorough and careful coding process are all measures included to support the cogency of the analysis and to minimize incorrect representations. These elements also relate to the analytical process (for instance the attentiveness towards the relationship between the whole life story and its various parts) and the issue of validity, at large. Needless to say, representation also involves a respectful and conscientious treatment of each interview and the set of data material in general, but in the end, the analysis still reflect my selection, presentation and interpretation of the interviews.

A.3.4 Sensitive and Emotional Matters

The life stories narrated and conveyed in this book express to various extents, intimate and emotional issues, including personal experiences entailing loss, grief and sorrow. Several ethical issues arise in this regard; one issue relates to the handling and representation of very personal and intimate stories and involve the general question on 'how do we deal with painful, sensitive and emotional issues?' as posed by Merrill and West (2009, p. 208). The question does not yield any straightforward answers but I regard this as a matter of treating and conveying life stories/specific elements in a respectful and conscientious way, taking into account individual boundaries. Another issue relates to the specific interview interaction and the ethically subjective assessment in the specific dialogue of 'what might we choose not to ask, and why?' (Merrill and West, 2009, p. 208). Such an assessment relies on the researcher's success with establishing a setting of trust and requires the researcher to exhibit sensitivity towards potential emotional issues. I agree with Merrill and West when they state that

> ...fundamentally, being ethical stems from treating people as full human beings: knowing, creative subjects in their own right rather than repositories of 'data' to be extracted and understood by us alone.
>
> (2009, p. 207)

A.4 Supplementary Data Sources and Data Collection

In addition to the primary method of biographical narrative research, the study applies a number of methods to support and inform the analysis of solo motherhood and the formation of donor-conceived families.

A.4.1 Expert Interviews

A limited number of semi-structured expert interviews have been performed to obtain more general data on developments in the proliferation of medically assisted reproduction, course of treatment and particular issues pertaining to single women/solo mothers undergoing fertility treatment. As practicians, they offer unique and professional insights into the field. I conducted expert interviews with the following three experts: Professor Lone Schmidt is located at the Department of Public Health at the University of Copenhagen. She is an expert within research areas such as reproductive health, assisted reproduction and solo motherhood, among others. Maria Salomon is a nurse and researcher at the Fertility Clinic, Rigshospitalet. She has furthermore initiated the fertility clinic's implementation of network groups for single women embarking upon solo motherhood in which she partly participates. Karin Erb is laboratory Director at the Fertility Clinic at Odense University, and is former Chairperson of the National Danish Fertility Society. The Society collects annual data on ART and IUI treatments initiated nationally and Karin holds main responsibility for the figures/statistics established. The interviews were conducted as semi-structured interviews with a fairly comprehensive interview guide that was adapted to the individual expert interview to explore the specific fields of expertise. The interviews have been thematically coded in NVivo and have both informed the design of the biographical narrative interviews and the analysis in general.

A.4.2 Observation Study

A minor observation study at a public fertility clinic was conducted in order to gain insight in the entire process of fertility treatment; from preliminary medicals, through to the actual process of insemination/IVF with donor semen (IUI-D, IVF-D) and to the actual 'laboratory practices'. The purpose with this small-scale field work was to experience the clinical setting first hand as an observer, to witness the health professionals' use of the technologies on site and to be able, to a greater extent, to situate and contextualize the women's personal accounts. I spent 2 days at the clinic in august 2015, during which time I mainly shadowed (to borrow an expression from Charis Thompson, 2005, p. 15) three chief physicians. I attended a number of key procedures: the initial nurse consultation, ultrasound scans (two of which were with single women), egg retrieval and embryo transfer (see Chapter 5 for details). I also visited the laboratory where I observed images of fertilized oocytes dividing into blastocysts, along with a sperm quality test. The short duration of my time at the clinic does not allow for any far-reaching or exhaustive conclusions regarding patient and staff behaviour or this particular social setting in general. It did however allow me to achieve the study objectives of witnessing different fertility procedures/practices, experiencing the particular atmosphere/setting and additionally via short, informal conversations with staff, to enquire about specific procedures/considerations/experiences of particular relevance for single women.

A.4.3 Interpretative Policy Analysis

Chapter 3 in the book provides a contextual understanding of the political and discursive environment of the governing of ARTs and aims to analyse possible transformations within our established conceptions of 'natural practices' in terms of family formation, procreation and motherhood. Through policy analysis/frame analysis, it is explored how policy positions are framed and legitimized in the Danish 2006/2007 parliamentary debates on equity of access to ARTs by using the theoretical concept of governmentality as a frame of reference. The analysis compares the 2006/2007 debates to the debates 10 years earlier (1996/1997) where access to assisted reproduction was restricted to heterosexual married women or women living in a 'marriage-like relationship'. The particulars regarding the application of frame analysis as a method, the specific parliamentary documents used, and the coding procedures applied, are described in detail in the chapter.

Appendix 2: Glossary on MAR

Assisted Reproductive Technology (ART): All interventions that include the in vitro handling of both human oocytes and sperm or of embryos for the purpose of reproduction. This includes, but is not limited to, IVF and embryo transfer ET, intracytoplasmic sperm injection ICSI, embryo biopsy, preimplantation genetic testing PGT, assisted hatching, gamete intrafallopian transfer GIFT, zygote intrafallopian transfer, gamete and embryocryopreservation, semen, oocyte and embryo donation, and gestational carrier cycles. Thus, ART does not, and ART-only registries do not, include assisted insemination using sperm from either a woman's partner or a sperm donor. (See broader term, medically assisted reproduction, MAR.)

Cross border reproductive care: The provision of reproductive health services in a different jurisdiction or outside of a recognized national border within which the person or persons legally reside.

Cryopreservation: The process of slow freezing or vitrification to preserve biological material (e.g. gametes, zygotes, cleavage-stage embryos, blastocysts or gonadal tissue) at extreme low temperature.

Embryo: The biological organism resulting from the development of the zygote, until eight completed weeks after fertilization, equivalent to 10 weeks of gestational age.

Embryo donation (for reproduction): An ART cycle, which consists of the transfer of an embryo to the uterus or fallopian tube of a female recipient, resulting from gametes that did not originate from the female recipient or from her male partner, if present.

Embryo transfer (ET): Placement into the uterus of an embryo at any embryonic stage from day 1 to day 7 after IVF or ICSI. Embryos from day 1 to day three can also be transferred into the fallopian tube.

Endometriosis: A disease characterized by the presence of endometrium-like epithelium and stroma outside the endometrium and myometrium. Intrapelvic endometriosis can be located superficially on

Lived Realities of Solo Motherhood, Donor Conception
and Medically Assisted Reproduction, 199–200
Copyright © 2021 Tine Ravn
Published under exclusive licence by Emerald Publishing Limited
doi:10.1108/978-1-83909-115-520211012

the peritoneum (peritoneal endometriosis), can extend 5 mm or more beneath the peritoneum (deep endometriosis) or can be present as an ovarian endometriotic cyst (endometrioma).

Fertilization: A sequence of biological processes initiated by entry of a spermatozoon into a mature oocyte followed by formation of the pronuclei.

Frozen/thawed embryo transfer cycle (FET): An ART procedure in which cycle monitoring is carried out with the intention of transferring to a woman, frozen/thawed or vitrified/warmed embryo(s)/ blastocyst(s). Note: A FET cycle is initiated when specific medication is provided or cycle monitoring is started in the female recipient with the intention to transfer an embryo.

In vitro fertilization (IVF): A sequence of procedures that involves extracorporeal fertilization of gametes. It includes conventional in vitro insemination and ICSI.

Infertility: A disease characterized by the failure to establish a clinical pregnancy after 12 months of regular, unprotected sexual intercourse or due to an impairment of a person's capacity to reproduce either as an individual or with his/her partner. Fertility interventions may be initiated in less than 1 year based on medical, sexual and reproductive history, age, physical findings and diagnostic testing. Infertility is a disease, which generates disability as an impairment of function.

Intra-cytoplasmic sperm injection (ICSI): Procedure in which a single spermatozoon is injected into the oocyte cytoplasm.

Intra-uterine insemination: A procedure in which laboratory processed sperm are placed in the uterus to attempt a pregnancy.

Medically assisted reproduction (MAR): Reproduction brought about through various interventions, procedures, surgeries and technologies to treat different forms of fertility impairment and infertility. These include ovulation induction, ovarian stimulation, ovulation triggering, all ART procedures, uterine transplantation and intra-uterine, intracervical and intravaginal insemination with semen of husband/ partner or donor.

Source: The terms and definitions are directly reproduced from the following reference, as they are internationally acknowledged as the standard MAR glossary within scientific and medical communities: Zegers-Hochschild, F. et al. (2017). The International Glossary on Infertility and Fertility Care, 2017. *Human Reproduction*, 32(9), pp. 1786–1801.

References

Adrian, S. 2006. *Nye skabelsesberetninger om æg, sæd og embryoner.* PhD. Linköping Studies in Arts and Science No. 370. Linköpings universitet: Institutionen för Tema.

Adrian, S.W. 2014. Assisteret befrugtning, en feministisk teoretisk udfordring? *Kvinder, Køn and Forskning,* 3, 54–68.

Albæk, E., Green-Pedersen, C. and Larsen, L.T. 2012. Morality issues in Denmark, policies without politics. In *Morality Politics in Western Europe: Parties, Agendas and Policy Choices,* Eds I. Engeli, C. Green-Pedersen and L.T. Larsen, pp. 137–160, London, Palgrave Macmillan.

Almeling, R. 2009. Gender and the value of bodily goods: commodification in egg and sperm donation, *Law and Contemporary Problems,* 72(3), 37–58.

Almeling, R. and Willey, I.L. 2017. Same medicine, different reasons: comparing women's bodily experiences of producing egss for pregnancy or for profit, *Social Science & Medicine,* 188, 21–29.

Andersen, H. 2005. Diskursanalyse. In *Leksikon i sociologi,* Eds H. Andersen, et al., Copenhagen, Akademisk Forlag.

Andersen, N.A., Ingerslev, H.J. and Humaidan, P.S. 2012. Fra skepsis til accept af assisteret befrugtning, *Ugeskrift for Læger,* 174(41), 2438.

Andreassen, R. 2018. Introduction. Motherhood and the Web 2.0. In *Mediated Kinship: Gender, Race and Sexuality in Donor Families,* Ed. R. Andreassen, London, Routledge.

Andrews, M. 2012. What is narrative interviewing? In *NCRM Research Methods Festival 2012, 2–5 July 2012,* Oxford, St. Catherine's College (Unpublished).

Andrews, M., Squire, C. and Tamboukou, M. 2013. Introduction: what is narrative research? In *Doing Narrative Research,* Eds M. Andrews, C. Squire and M. Tamboukou, 2nd ed., Los Angeles, CA, SAGE.

Antoft, R. and Thomsen, T.L. 2005. Når livsfortællinger bliver en sociologisk metode – en introduktion til det biografisk narrative interview. In *Liv, fortælling og tekst – Strejftog i kvalitativ sociologi,* Eds M.H. Jacobsen, S. Kristiansen and A. Prieur, Aalborg, Aalborg Universitetsforlag.

Almeling, R. 2011. *Sex Cells. The Medical Market for Eggs and Sperm,* Berkeley, University of California Press.

Almeling, R. 2014. Kinship and the market for sex cells. In *Presentation presented at the International Critical Kinship Conference,* Odense, Denmark, October 9–10, 2014.

Bacchi, C. 2009. The issue of intentionality in frame theory: the need for reflexive framing. In *The Discursive Politics of Gender Equality: Stretching, Bending and Policymaking,* Eds E. Lombardo, P. Meier and M. Verloo, pp. 19–35, Abingdon, Routledge.

Baía, I., de Freitas, C. and Silva, S. 2021. Priority of access to fertility treatments based on sexual orientation and marital status: the views of gamete donors and recipients. *Sexuality Research and Social Policy,* 18, 368–376.

Bajekal, N. 2019. Why so many women travel to Denmark for fertility treatments, *Time,* 3 January. Available at: https://time.com/5491636/denmark-ivf-storkklinik-fertility/

Baldwin, K. 2019. Introduction. In *Egg Freezing, Fertility and Reproductive Choice: Negotiating Responsibility, Hope and Modern Motherhood*, Ed. K. Baldwin, Bingley, Emerald Publishing Limited.

Balling, G. and Lippert-Rasmussen, K. 2006. Introduktion. In *Det menneskelige eksperiment: Om menneskesyn og moderne bioteknologi*, Eds G. Balling and K. Lippert-Rasmussen, pp. 9–22, Copenhagen, Museum Tusculanums Forlag.

Bauchspies, W.K., Croissant, J. and Revisto, S. 2006. *Science, Technology, and Society. A Sociological Approach*, Malden, MA, Blackwell Publishing.

Beck, U. and Beck-Gernsheim, E. 2001. *Individualization*, London, Sage Publications.

Beck-Gernsheim, E. 2002. *Reinventing the Family*, Cambridge, Polity Press.

Becker, G. 2000. *The Elusive Embryo: How Women and Men Approach New Reproductive Technologies*. [e-book], Berkeley, CA, University of California Press.

Birenbaum-Carmeli, D. 2016. Thirty-five years of assisted reproductive technologies in Israel, *Reproductive BioMedicine & Society Online*, 2, 16–23.

Blake, L., Casey, P., Jadva, V. and Golombok, S. 2013. 'I was quite amazed': donor conception and parent–child relationships from the child's perspective, *Children & Society*, 28(6), 425–437.

Blyth, E. and Frith, L. 2009. Donor-conceived people's access to genetic and biographical history: an analysis of provisions in different jurisdictions permitting disclosure of donor identity, *International Journal of Law, Policy and the Family*, 23(2), 174–191.

Blyth, E. and Landau, R. 2003. Introduction. In *Third Party Assisted Conceptions Across Cultures. Social, Legal and Ethical Perspectives*, Eds E. Blyth and R. Landau, pp.7–21, New York, Jessica Kingley Publishers.

Bo, I.G. 2005. At sætte tavsheder i tale – fortolkning og forståelse I det kvalitative forskningsinterview. In *Liv, fortælling og tekst – Strejftog i kvalitativ sociologi*, Eds M.H. Jacobsen, S. Kristiansen and A. Prieur, Aalborg, Aalborg Universitetsforlag.

Bock, J. 2000. Emergent and reconfigured forms of family life: doing the right thing? Single mothers by choice and the struggle for legitimacy, *Gender & Society*, 14(1), 62–86.

Borchhorst, A. and Siim, B. 2008. Women-friendly policies and state feminism: theorizing Scandinavian gender equality, *Feminist Theory*, 9(2), 207–244.

Bourdieu, P. and Wacquant, L.J.D. 1996. *Refleksiv sociologi*, København, Hans Reitzels Forlag.

Brake, E. and Millum, J. 2012. Parenthood and procreation. In *The Stanford Encyclopedia of Philosophy*, Ed. E.N. Zalta, Spring 2012 Edition. [online], Stanford, CA, The Metaphysics Lab, Center for the Study of Language and Information, Stanford University. Available at: http://plato.stanford.edu/archives/spr2012/entries/parenthood/

Brejnholt, K. 2013. *Her er familien Danmark*. [pdf], Copenhagen, Statistics Denmark. Available at: www.dst.dk/-/media/Kontorer/15-Kundecenter/Statistisk-Perspektiv-8/p8art1.pdf

Brubaker, R. and Cooper, F. 2000. Beyond "identity", *Theory and Society*, 29, 1–47. The Netherlands: Kluwer Academic Publishers.

Bruner, J. 2004. Life as Narrative. *Social Research*, 71(3), 691–710.

Bryld, M. 2001. The infertility clinic and the birth of the lesbian, *European Journal of Women's Studies*, 8(3), 299–312.

Bryld, M. and Lykke, N. 2000. Mellem kunstig befrugtning og naturlig intelligens: Om skiftende betydninger af køn og kvalitet, *Kvinder, Køn and Forskning*, 9(2), 16–26.

Budgeon, S. and Roseneil, S. 2004. Editors' introduction: beyond the conventional family. *Current Sociology*, 52(2), 127–134. doi: 10.1177/0011392104041797

Butler, J. 1988. Performative acts and gender constitution: an essay in phenomenology and feminist theory, *Theatre Journal*, 40(4), 519–531.

Butler, J. 1993. *Bodies that Matter. On the Discursive Limits of "Sex"*, London, Routledge.

Butler, J. 1999 [1990]. *Gender Trouble. Feminism and the Subversion of Identity*, London, Routledge.

Butler, J. (with Olsen, G. and Worsham, L.) 2004. Changing the subject: Judith Butler's politics of radical resignification. In *The Judith Butler Reader*, Ed. S. Salih with J. Butler, pp. 325–356, Oxford, Blackwell.

Calhaz-Jorge, C., et al. 2020. Survey on ART and IUI: legislation, regulation, funding and registries in European countries, *Human Reproduction Open*, 2020, 1–15.

Carsten, J. 2000. Introduction: cultures of relatedness. In *Cultures of Relatedness. New Approaches to the Study of Kinship*, Ed. J. Carsten, Cambridge, Cambridge University Press.

Carsten, J. 2004. *After Kinship*, Cambridge, Cambridge University Press.

Chamberlayne, P., Bornat, J., and Wengraf, T. 2000. Introduction: the biographical turn. In *The Turn to Biographical Methods in Social Science: Comparative Issues and Examples*, Eds P. Chamberlayne, J. Bornat and T. Wengraf, pp. 1–30, London, Routledge.

Chan, R.W., et al. 1998. Psychosocial adjustment among children conceived via donor insemination by lesbian and heterosexual mothers. *Child Development*, 69(2), 443–457.

Charmaz, K. 2006. *Constructing Grounded Theory: A Practical Guide through Qualitative Analysis*, London; Thousand Oaks; New Delhi, SAGE.

Chase, S.E. 2005. Narrative inquiry: multiple lenses, approaches, voices. In *The SAGE Handbook of Qualitative Research*, Eds N. Denzin and Y.S. Lincoln, pp. 651–679, Thousand Oaks, CA, Sage Publications.

Christiansen, P.O. 2007. Indledning. In *En rigtig familie – mellem nye og gamle idealer*, Eds L. Andersen and P.O. Christiansen, København, C. A. Reitzels Forlag.

Cooper, M. and Waldby, C. 2014. *Clinical Labor. Tissue Donors and Research Subjects in the Global Economy*, Durham, NC, Duke University Press.

Corbally, M. and O'Neill, C.S. 2014. An introduction to the biographical narrative interpretive method, *Nurse Researcher*, 21(5), 34–39.

Courduriés, J. and Herbrand, C. 2014. Gender, kinship and assisted reproductive technologies: future directions after 30 years of research, *Enfances, Familles, Générations*, 21, 1–27.

Cryos International. 2019. *Fertility trend: People who are involuntary childless request personal Knowledge about the sperm donor. News Letter*. Available at: https://www.cryosinternational.com/content/da-dk/sysglobalassets/cryos-denmark/shared-dk/press/pressemeddelelser-dk/fertilitetstrend-barnloese-efterspoerger-personlig-viden-om-saeddonorer.pdf

Cussins, C. 1996. Ontological choreography: agency through objectification in infertility clinics, *Social Studies of Science*, 26(3), 575–610.

Cutas, D. and Chan, S. 2012. Introduction: perspectives on private and family life. In *Families – beyond the Nuclear Ideal*, Eds D. Cutas and S. Chan, pp. 1–12, London, Bloomsbury Academic.

Dang, V.Q., et al. 2019. The effectiveness of ICSI versus conventional IVF in couples with non-male factor infertility: study protocol for a randomised controlled trial, *Human Reproduction Open*, 2019(2), 1–6.

Danish Fertility Society. 2020a. *Results for 2019*, Copenhagen, Danish Fertility Society. Available at: http://www.fertilitetsselskab.dk/

Danish Fertility Society. 2020b. *Results for 2018*. Copenhagen: Danish Fertility Society. Available at: http://www.fertilitetsselskab.dk/

Danish Fertility Society. 2020c. *Results for 2013*. Copenhagen: Danish Fertility Society. Available at: http://www.fertilitetsselskab.dk/

Danish Patient Safety Authority. 2020. Legislative material for medically assisted reproduction. Available at: https://stps.dk/da/ansvar-og-retningslinjer/vejledning/assisteret-reproduktion/lovmateriale/

Denzin, N.K. 1989. *Interpretive Biography*, London, Sage Publications.

Edwards, J. 2009. Introduction: the matter in kinship. In *European Kinship in the Age of Biotechnology*, Eds J. Edwards and C. Salazar, pp. 1–19, Oxford, Berghahn Books.

Ellingsæter, A.L., Jensen, A. and Lie, M. 2013. *The Social Meaning of Children and Fertility Change in Europe*, Abingdon, Routledge.

Engeli, I. 2009. The challenges of abortion and assisted reproductive technologies policies in Europe. *Comparative European Politics*, 7(1), 56–74.

Engeli, I. and Varone, F. 2011. Governing morality issues through procedural policies. *Swiss Political Science Review*, 17(3), 239–258.

Ernst, E., et al. 2020. Fertility treatment. *Sundhed.dk*. Available at: https://www.sundhed.dk/sundhedsfaglig/information-til-praksis/midtjylland/almen-praksis/patientforloeb/forloebsbeskrivelser/w-svangerskab-foedsel-svangerskabsforebyggelse/fertilitetsbehandling/

ESHRE. 2012. Higher levels of public reimbursement positively influence national birth rates and reduce unmet needs in subfertile populations. [press release] 2 July 2012. Available at: https://www.eshre.eu/Press-Room/Press-releases/Press-releases-ESHRE-2012/ART-reimbursement.aspx

ESHRE. 2016. Three in four women starting fertility treatment will have a baby within five years. [online]. Available at: http://www.eshre2016.eu/Media/Press-releases_/Malchau.aspx

ESHRE. 2017. Regulation and legislation in assisted reproduction. [online]. Available at: file:///C:/Users/au311243/AppData/Local/Temp/2%20Regulation.pdf

ESHRE. 2020. *ART fact sheet*. [online]. Available at: https://www.eshre.eu/Press-Room/Resources

Esping-Andersen, G. 2009. *The Incomplete Revolution: Adapting Welfare States to Women's New Roles*, Cambridge, Polity Press.

Flick, U. 2009. *An Introduction to Qualitative Research*, 4th ed., London, SAGE.

Foucault, M. 1983. The subject and power. In *Michel Foucault: Beyond Structuralism and Hermeneutics*, Eds H.L. Dreyfus and P. Rabinow, pp. 208–226, Chicago, IL, The University of Chicago Press.

Foucault, M. 1994. *Viljen til viden: Seksualitetens historie 1*, Frederiksberg, Det Lille Forlag.

Franklin, S. 1993. Essentialism, which essentialism? Some implications of reproductive and genetic techno-science. In *If You Seduce a Straight Person, Can You Make Them Gay? Issues in Biological Essentialism Versus Social Constructionism in Gay and Lesbian Identities*, Eds J.P. De Cecco and J.P. Elia, pp. 27–39, New York, NY: The Haworth Press.

Franklin, S. 1997. *Embodied Progress. A Cultural Account of Assisted Conception*, New York, NY, Routledge.

Franklin, S. 2001. Biologization revisited: kinship theory in the context of the new biologies. In *Relative Values: Reconfiguring Kinship Studies*, Eds S. Franklin and S. McKinnon, pp. 302–325, London: Duke University Press.

Franklin, S. 2008. Reimagining the facts of life, *Soundings*, 40(3), 147–156.

Franklin, S. 2013a. *Biological Relatives: IVF, Stem Cells, and the Future of Kinship*, Durham, NC, Duke University Press.

Franklin, S. 2013b. Transforming kinship. In *eLS*, Chichester, Wiley.

Franklin, S. and Lock, M. 2003. Animation and cessation: the remaking of life and death. In *Remaking Life and Death: Toward an Anthropology of the Biosciences*, Eds S. Franklin and M. Lock, Oxford, James Currey.

Franklin, S. and McKinnon, S. 2001. Relative values: reconfiguring kinship studies. In *Relative Values: Reconfiguring Kinship Studies*, Eds S. Franklin and S. McKinnon, pp. 1–25, London, Duke University Press.

Frederiksen, M.E. 2010. *Solomødre – Når enlige kvinder vælger at danne familie ved hjælp af donor-insemination*. Master's thesis, Institute for Public Health, University of Copenhagen.

Frederiksen, M.E, Christensen, U., Tjørnhøj-Thomsen, T. and Schmidt, L. 2011. Solo mother by donor – the plan B of motherhood. A perspective on person-centered reproductive medicine, *International Journal of Person Centered Medicine*, 1(4), 800–807.

Freeman, T. 2014. Introduction. In *Relatedness in Assisted Reproduction: Families, Origins and Identities*, Eds T. Freeman, S. Graham, F. Ebtehaj and M. Richards, pp. 1–20, Cambridge, Cambridge University Press.

Frith, L. 2020. From the nuclear family towards family network models through ART. Presentation given at an ESHRE workshop on "Moving on from Individual Connections to Networks: New Challenges in Donor Conception" in Leuven, Belgium (February 2020).

Frost, R. 1949. *Complete Poems of Robert Frost*, New York, NY, Henry Holt and Company.

Fujii, L.A. 2012. Research ethics 101: dilemmas and responsibilities, *PS: Political Science & Politics*, 45(4), 717–723.

Gamble, N. 2009. Considering the need for a father: the role of clinicians in safeguarding family values in UK fertility treatment, *Ethnics, Bioscience and Life*, 4(2), 15–18.

Giddens, A. 1991. *Modernity and Self-Identity: Self and Society in the Late Modern Age*, Stanford, CA, Stanford University Press.

Gillis, J. 1996. *A World of Their Own Making: Myth, Ritual, and the Quest for Family Values*, New York, NY, Basic Books.

Ginsburg, F.D. 1989. *Contested Lives. The Abortion Debate in an American Community*, Berkeley, University of California Press.

Glaser, B.G. 1998. Forcing the data. In *Doing Grounded Theory: Issues and Discussions*, Ed. B.G. Glaser, Mill Valley, CA, The Sociology Press.

Goffman, E. 1992. *Vore rollespil i hverdagen*, Copenhagen, Hans Reitzels Forlag.

Goffman, E. 2009. *Stigma*, 2nd ed., Copenhagen, Samfundslitteratur.

Golombok, S. 2012. Families created by reproductive donation: issues and research, *Child Development Perspectives*, 7(1), 61–65.

Golombok, S. 2013. *Happy Families. Focus on Reproduction*, European Society of Human Reproduction and Embryology, January 2013, pp. 30–34.

Golombok, S. 2015. *Modern Families: Parents and Children in New Family Forms*, Cambridge, Cambridge University Press.

Golombok, S. 2020. Single mothers by choice: 'different shapes'. In *We Are Family. What Really Matters for Parents and Children*, Ed. S. Golombok, London, Scribe Publications.

Golombok, S. and Badger, S. 2010. Children raised in mother-headed families from infancy: a follow-up of children of lesbian and single heterosexual mothers, at early adulthood, *Human Reproduction*, 25(1), 150–157.

Golombok, S., Tasker, F. and Murray, C. 1997. Children raised in fatherless families from infancy: family relationships and the socio-emotional development of children of lesbian and single heterosexual mothers, *Journal of Child Psychology and Psychiatry*, 38(7), 783–792.

Golombok, S., Zadeh, S., Freeman, T., Lysons, J. and Foley, S. 2020. Single mothers by choice: parenting and child adjustment in middle childhood, *Journal of Family Psychology*. Advance online publication. doi:10.1037/fam0000797

Golombok, S., Zadeh, S, Imrie, S. Smith, V. and Freeman, T. 2016. Single mothers by choice: mother-child relationships and children's psychological adjustment, *Journal of Family Psychology*, 30(4), 409–418.

Grace, V.M., Daniels, K. and Gillett, W. 2008. The donor, the father, and the imaginary constitution of the family: parents' constructions in the case of donor insemination, *Social Science and Medicine*, 66(2), 301–314.

Graham, S. 2012. Choosing single motherhood - single women negotiating the nuclear family ideal. In *Families – beyond the Nuclear Ideal*, Eds D. Cutas and S. Chan, London, Bloomsbury Academic. Cp. 7.

Graham, S. 2013. *Imagined Futures: Experiences and Decision-Making of Single Women Embarking upon Motherhood through Sperm Donation*. PhD, University of Cambridge.

Graham, S. 2014. Stories of an absent 'father': single women negotiating relatedness through donor profiles. In *Relatedness in Assisted Reproduction: Families, Origins and Identities*, Eds T. Freeman, S. Graham, F. Ebtehaj and M. Richards, pp. 212–231, Cambridge, Cambridge University Press.

Graham, S. 2018. Being a 'good' parent: single women reflecting upon 'selfishness' and 'risk' when pursuing motherhood through sperm donation, *Anthropology & Medicine*, 25(3), 249–264. doi: 10.1080/13648470.2017.1326757

Graham, S. and Braverman, A. 2012. ARTs and the single parent. In *Reproductive Donation: Practice, Policy and Bioethics*, Eds M. Richards, G. Pennings and J.B. Appleby, pp. 189–210, Cambridge, Cambridge University Press.

Graham, S. and Ravn, T. 2016. Ideals versus realities: exploring methodological influences on eliciting narratives of solo mothers. Presentation presented to the session 'Social Studies of Reproduction: techniques, methods and reflexive moments' at the ISA RC33 Methodology Conference, Leicester, September 2015.

Grill, E.A. 2005. Treating single mothers by choice. In *Frozen Dreams: Psychodynamic Dimensions of Infertility and Assisted Reproduction*, Eds A. Rosen and J. Rosen, Hillsdale, NJ, The Analytic Press.

Haimes, E. and Daniels, K. 1998. International social sciences perspectives: an introduction. In *Donor Insemination. International Social Science Perspectives*, Eds E. Haimes and K. Danieks, pp. 1–7, Cambridge, Cambridge University Press.

Haraway, D. 1988. Situated knowledges: the science question in feminism and the privilege of partial perspective, *Feminist Studies*, 14(3), 575–599.

Haraway, D. 2000. *How Like a Leaf. An Interview with Thyrza Nichols Goodeve*, New York, NY, Routledge.

Haraway, D. 2004a. The promises of monsters: a regenerative politics for inappropriate/d others. In *The Haraway Reader*, Ed. D. Haraway, pp. 63–124, London, Routledge.

Haraway, D. with Lykke, N., Markussen, R. and Olesen, F. 2004b [2000]. Cyborgs, coytes, and dogs: a kinship of feminist figurations and there are always more things going on than you thought! Methodologies as thinking technologies. An interview with Donna Haraway. In *The Haraway Reader*, Ed. D. Haraway, pp. 321–343, London, Routledge.

Hanson, A.F. 2001. Donor insemination: eugenic and feminist implications, *Medical Anthropology Quaterly*, 15(3), 287–311.

Hauskeller, C., et al. 2013. Genetics and the sociology of identity, *Sociology*, 47(5), 875–886.

Heinz, W.R. and Krüger, H. 2001. Life course: innovations and challenges for social research, *Current Sociology*, 49(2), 29–45.

HelseNorge. 2020. Involuntary childlessness and assisted reproduction. Available at: https://www.helsenorge.no/en/refusjon-og-stotteordninger/involuntary-childlessness-and-assisted-reproduction/

Herrmann, J.R. 2018. Assisted reproduction in Denmark. Available at SSRN: https://ssrn.com/abstract=3198538

Hertz, R. 2002. The father as an idea: a challenge to kinship boundaries by single mothers, *Symbolic Interaction*, 25(1), 1–31.

Hertz, R. 2006. Talking about "doing" family, *Journal of Marriage and Family*, 68(4), 796–799.

Hertz, R. 2021. Single mothers as bricoleurs: crafting embryos and kin, *Journal of Family Issues*, 42(1), 1–30.

Hertz, R. and Nelson, M.K. 2019. *Random Families. Genetic Strangers, Sperm Donor Siblings, and the Creation of New Kin*, Oxford, Oxford University Press.

Hoerning, E.M. 1996. *Life Course and Biography: Approaches and Methods*, Aalborg University, Department of Development and Planning, Series no. 199, December, 1996.

Hoerning, E.M. 2001. Fra biografisk metode til biografiforskning, *Dansk Sociologi*, 12(3), 117–125.

Hoffmann-Hansen, H. 2006. Sådan fik lesbiske og enlige adgang til kunstig befrugtning, *Kristeligt Dagblad*. [online] 3 June. Available at: http://www.etik.dk/kunstig-befrugtning/s%C3%A5dan-fik-lesbiske-og-enlige-adgang-til-kunstig-befrugtning

Horsdal, M. 2012. *Telling Lives. Exploring Dimensions of Narratives*, London; New York, NY, Routledge.

Højgaard, L. 2012. Judith Butler. Det performative køn og de sociale kategoriers dekonstruktion. In *Samfundsteori og Samtidsdiagnose. En Introduktion til Sytten Nyere Samfundstænkere for det Pædagogiske Felt*, Eds M.H. Jacobsen and A. Petersen, pp. 280–294, København, Forlaget Unge Pædagoger.

IFFS (The International Federation of Fertility Societies). 2019. IFFS Surveillance 2019. *Global Reproductive Health (2019)*, 4, e29.

Inhorn, M.C. and Birenbaum-Carmeli, D. 2008. Assisted reproductive technologies and culture change, *Annual Review of Anthropology*, 37(1), 177–196.

Jadva, V., et al. 2009a. 'Mom by choice, single by life's circumstance...' Findings from a large scale survey of the experiences of single mothers by choice, *Human Fertility*, 12(4), 175–184.

Jadva, V., et al. 2009b. The experiences of adolescents and adults conceived by sperm donation: comparisons by age of disclosure and family type, *Human Reproduction*, 24(8), 1909–1919.

Jenkins, R. 2008. *Social Identity*, 3rd ed., London, Routledge.

Jenny, J.G. 2013. Europeanizing reproduction: reproductive technologies in Europe and Scandinavia, *NORA - Nordic Journal of Feminist and Gender Research*, 21(3), 236–242. doi: 10.1080/08038740.2013.826276

Jones, S. 2007. Exercising agency, becoming a single mother, *Marriage and Family Review*, 42(4), 35–61.

Järvinen, M. 2005. Interview i en interaktionistisk begrebsramme. In *Kvalitative metoder i et interaktionistisk perspektiv*, Eds N. Mik-Meyer and M. Järvinen, pp. 27–48, København, Hans Reitzels Forlag.

Keller, E.F. 2010. *The Mirage of Space between Nature and Nurture*, Durham, NC; London, Duke University Press.

Kennedy, S. and Ruggles, S. 2014. Breaking up is hard to count: the rise of divorce in the United States, 1980-2010, *Demography*, 51, 587–598.

Klitzman, R. 2016. Deciding how many embryos to transfer: ongoing challenges and dilemmas, *Reproductive Biomedicine & Society Online*, 3, 1–15.

Knecht, M., Klotz, M. and Beck, S. 2012. Introduction. In *Reproductive Technologies as Global Form: Ethnographies of Knowledge, Practices, and Transnational Encounters*, Eds M. Knecht, M. Klotz and S. Beck, Frankfurt, Campus Verlag.

Knudsen, L.B. 2009. *Fertilitet og familiedannelse – et felt mellem valg og skæbne*. Sociologisk Arbejdspapir, CASTOR, 26, Tiltrædelsesforelæsning ved Aalborg Universitet 2008.

Knudsen, L.B. (2014). Familien i Danmark. In *Pædagogisk sociologi*, Eds H. Dorf and J. Rasmussen, pp. 165–186, Copenhagen, Hans Reitzels Forlag.

Konrad, M. 1998. Ova donation and symbols of substance: some variations on the theme of sex, gender and the partible body, *Journal of the Royal Anthropological Institute*, 4(4), 643–667.

Kooli, C. 2019. Review of assisted reproduction techniques, laws, and regulations in Muslim countries, *Middle East Fertility Society Journal*, 24(8), 1–15.

Kroløkke, C., et al. 2019. Introduction. In *The Cryopolitics of Reproduction on Ice: A New Scandinavian Ice Age*, Eds C. Kroløkke, et al., pp. 1–18, Bingley, Emerald Publishing Limited.

Kushnir, V.A., et al. 2017. Systematic review of worldwide trends in assisted reproductive technology 2004–2013. *Reproductive biology and endocrinology: RB&E*, 15(1), 6. doi: 10.1186/s12958-016-0225-2

Lampic, C., Skoog Svanberg, A. and Sydsjö, G. 2014. Attitudes towards disclosure and relationship to donor offspring among a national cohort of identity-release oocyte and sperm donors, *Human Reproduction*, 29(9), 1978–1986.

Landau, R., et al. 2008. A child of "hers": older single mothers and their children conceived through IVF with both egg and sperm donation, *Fertility and Sterility*, 90(3), 576–583.

Laws, D. and Rein, M. 2003. Reframing practice. In *Deliberative Policy Analysis: Understanding Governance in the Network Society*, Eds M. Hajer and H. Wagenaar, pp. 172–208, Cambridge, Cambridge University Press.

Leiblum, S.R., et al. 1995. Non-traditional mothers: single heterosexual/lesbian women and lesbian couples electing motherhood via donor insemination, *Journal of Psychosomatic Obstetrics and Gynaecology*, 16, 11–20.

Lemke, T. 2009. *Biopolitik: En introduktion*, Copenhagen, Hans Reitzels Forlag.

Lesnik-Oberstein, K. 2008. *On Having an Own Child. Reproductive Tehnologies and the Cultural Construction of Childhod*, London, Karnac Books.

Levine, N.E. 2008. Alternative kinship, marriage, and reproduction, *Annual Review of Anthropology*, 37, 375–389.

Lie, M. 2002. Science as father? Sex and gender in the age of reproductive technologies, *European Journal of Women's Studies*, 9(4), 381–399.

Lock, M. and Nguyen, V. 2010. Kinship, infertility and assisted reproduction. In *An Anthropology of Biomedicine*, Eds M. Lock and V. Nguyen, pp. 254–277, Chichester, Wiley-Blackwell.

Lykke, N. 2008. Feminist cultural studies of technoscience. In *Bits of Life: Feminism at the Intersections of Media, Biosci-ence, and Technology*, Eds A. Smelik and N. Lykke, pp. 3–15, Seattle, WA, University of Washington Press.

Lykke, N. 2010. The timeliness of post-constructionisme, *NORA – Nordic Journal of Feminist and Gender Research*, 18(2), 131–136.

Lykke, N. and Bryld, M. 2006. Nye forplantningsteknologier og post-naturlig etik. In *Det menneskelige eksperiment: Om menneskesyn og moderne bioteknologi*, Eds G. Balling and K. Lippert-Rasmussen, pp. 23–49, Copenhagen, Museum Tusculanums Forlag.

MacCallum, F. and Golombok, S. 2004. Children raised in fatherless families from infancy: a follow-up of children of lesbian and single heterosexual mothers at early adolescence, *Journal of Child Psychology and Psychiatry*, 45(8), 1407–1419.

Malchau, S.S., et al. 2017. The long-term prognosis for live birth in couples initiating fertility treatments, *Human Reproduction*, 32(7), 1439–1449.

Malmquist, A., Björnstam, T. and Thunholm, A. 2019. Swedish children of single mothers by choice, and children of heterosexual couples, reflect on child conception and other paths to parenthood, *NORA - Nordic Journal of Feminist and Gender Research*, 27(3), 166–180.

Mannis, V.S. 1999. Single mothers by choice, *Familiy Relations*, 48(2), 121–128.

March, K. 2008. Motherhood, personal agency and breaching family norms. Book Review.

Markussen, R. and Gad, C. 2007. Feministisk STS. In *Introduktion til STS. Science, Technology, Society*, Eds P. Lauritsen, C.B. Jensen and F. Olesen, pp. 157–181, Copenhagen, Hans Reitzels Forlag.

Mason, J. 2008. Tangible affinities and the real life fascination of kinship, *Sociology*, 42(1), 29–45.

May, V. 2001. *Lone Motherhood in Finnish Women's Life Stories. Creating Meaning in a Narrative Context*. PhD, Åbo Academy University Press.

May, V. 2004. Meanings of lone motherhood within a broader family context, *The Sociological Review*, 52, 390–403.

May, V. 2015. Families and personal life: all change? In *Contemporary Sociology*, Ed. M. Holborn, pp. 471–472, Cambridge, Polity Press.

Mazor, A. 2004. Single motherhood via donor-insemination (Di): separation, absence, and family creation, *Contemporary Family Therapy*, 26(2), 199–215.

McAdams, D.P. and McLean, K.C. 2013. Narrative identity, *Current Directions in Psychological Science*, 22(3), 233–238.

McKinnon, S. 2015. Productive paradoxes of the assisted reproductive technologies in the context of the new kinship studies, *Journal of Family Issues*, 36(4), 461–479.

Melhuus, M. 2012. *Problems of Conception. Issues of Law, Biotechnology, Individuals and Kinship*, Oxford, Berghahn Books.

Memmi, D. 2003. Governing through speech: the new state administration of bodies, *Social Research*, 70(2), 645–658.

Merrill, B. and West, L. 2009. *Using Biographical Methods in Social Research*, London, SAGE.

Ministry of Health. 2015. *Vejledning om sundhedspersoners og vævscentres virksomhed og forpligtelser i forbindelse med assisteret reproduktion* [*Guidelines on Health Persons' and Tissue Centers' Business and Obligations in Relation to Assisted Reproduction*]. Instruction no. 9351 of 26 May 2015. [online], Copenhagen, Ministry of Health. Available at: https://www.retsinformation.dk/Forms/R0710.aspx?id=172755

Ministry of Health. 2019. Act on assisted reproduction in connection with treatment, diagnosis and research etc. No. 902 of august 23. Available at: https://www.retsinformation.dk/eli/lta/2019/902

Ministry of Health. 2020a. Double donation allowed for single women and couples. Availably at: https://www.sum.dk/Aktuelt/Nyheder/Sundhedspolitik/2007/December/Dobbeltdonation-tilladt-for-enlige-kvinder-og-par.aspx

Ministry of Health. 2020b. New political agreement lift the five-year storage limit for egg freezing. Available at: https://sum.dk/Aktuelt/Nyheder/Sundhedspolitik/2020/Oktober/Ny-politisk-aftale-ophaever5-aars-graense-for-nedfrysning-af-aeg.aspx

Mohr, S. 2015. Living kinship trouble: Danish sperm donors' narratives of relatedness, *Medical Anthropology*, 34 (5), 470-484.

Moore, D.S. 2011. Evelyn fox keller: the mirage of a space between nature and nurture, *Sci & Educ.* doi: 10.1007/s11191-011-9374-z

Morgan, D.H.G. 2011. Locating 'family practices', *Sociological Research Online*, 16(4), 1–9.

Mortelmans, D., et al. 2016. Introduction. A view through the family Kaleidoscope. In *Changing Family Dynamics and Demographic Evolution. The Family Kaleidoscope*, Eds D. Mortelmans, et al., Cheltenham, Edward Elgar Publishing.

Mukherjee, S. 2017. Genetics therapies: post human. In *The Gene. An Intimate Story*, Ed. S. Mukherjee, New York, NY, Scribner.

Murray, C. and Golombok, S. 2005a. Going it alone: solo mothers and their infants conceived by donor insemination, *American Journal of Orthopsychiatry*, 75(2), 242–253.

Murray, C. and Golombok, S. 2005b. Solo mothers and their donor insemination infants: follow-up at age 2 years, *Human Reproduction*, 20(6), 1655–2005.

Myong, L. 2014. Adoptionens tid er nu. *Information*, 6 January. [online]. Available at: https://www.information.dk/debat/2014/01/adoptionens-tid

National Health Service (NHS). 2020. Risks. IVF. Available at: https://www.nhs.uk/conditions/ivf/risks/

National Human Genome Research Institute. 2016. All about the human genome project (HGP). [online]. Available at: https://www.genome.gov/10001772/all-about-the-human-genome-project-hgp/

Nicholson, L. 1997. The myth of the traditional family. In *Feminism and Families*, Ed. H.L. Nelson, pp. 27–42, New York, NY, Routledge.

Nordqvist, P. 2017. Genetic thinking and everyday living: on family practices and family imaginaries, *The Sociological Review*. doi: 10.1177/0038026117711645

Nordqvist, P. and Smart, C. 2014. *Relative Strangers. Family Life, Genes and Donor Conception*, Hampshire, Palgrave Macmillan.

Norup, M. 2006. Reproduktionsteknologier nu og i den nære fremtid. In *Det menneskelige eksperiment: Om menneskesyn og moderne bioteknologi*, Eds G. Balling and K. Lippert-Rasmussen, pp. 51–74, Copenhagen, Museum Tusculanums Forlag.

Oehlenschläger, E. 2015. Flere sæddonorer siger ja til at møde deres donorbørn. *Politiken*, [online] June 13. Available at: http://politiken.dk/forbrugogliv/livsstil/familieliv/ECE2710495/flere-saeddonorer-siger-ja-til-at-moede-deres-donorboern/

Ottosen, H. 2005. Den Moderne Familie – og Familienetværks betydning, *Social Politik*, 5, 17–23.

Payne, J.G. 2016. Grammars of kinship: biological motherhood and assisted reproduction in the age of epigenetics. *Signs: Journal of Women in Culture and Society 2016*, 41(3). doi: 10.1086/684233

Payne, J.G. 2020. Third-party reproduction across borders through the lens of kinship grammars. Presentation given at an ESHRE workshop on "Moving on from Individual Connections to Networks: New Challenges in Donor Conception" in Leuven, Belgium (February 2020).

Perelli-Harris, B., et al. 2017. The rise in divorce and cohabitation: is there a link?. *Population and Development Review*, 43(2), 303–329. doi: 10.1111/padr.12063

Petersen, M.N. 2007. *Fra barnets tarv til ligestilling – en analyse og vurdering af diskurserne i Folketingets forhandlinger vedrørende lesbiske og enlige kvinders adgang til lægeassisteret kunstig befrugtning i en queerteoretisk optik*. Master's thesis, Copenhagen, Centre for Gender Studies, Faculty of the Humanities, University of Copenhagen.

Peterson, M.M. 2005. Assisted reproductive technologies and equity of access issues. *Journal of Medical Ethics*, 31(5), 280–285.

Phoenix, A. 2011. Psychosocial intersections: contextualising the accounts of adults who grew up in visibly ethnically different households. In *Framing Intersectionality: Debates on a Multi-faceted Concept in Gender Studies*, Eds H. Lutz, M.T.H. Vivar and L. Supik, pp. 137–154, Farnham: Ashgate Publishing.

Phoenix, A. 2013. Analysing narrative context. In *Doing Narrative Research*, Eds M. Andrews, C. Squire and M. Tamboukou, 2nd ed., Los Angeles, CA, SAGE.

Polkinghorne, D.E. 1988. *Narrative Knowing and the Human Sciences*, Albany, NY, State University of New York Press.

Präg, P. and Mills, M.C. 2017. Assisted reproductive technology in Europe: usage and regulation in the context of cross-border reproductive care. In *Childlessness in Europe: Contexts, Causes, and Consequences. Demographic Research Monographs (A Series of the Max Planck Institute for Demographic Research)*, Eds M. Kreyenfeld and D. Konietzka, Cham, Springer.

Ravn, T. and Sørensen, M.P. 2013. Interview with Elisabeth Beck-Gernsheim: family structures and family life in second modernity. [online] *Theory, Culture and Society*. Available at: http://www.theoryculturesociety.org/interview-with-elisabeth-beck-gernsheim-on-individualization/

Rein, M. and Schön, D. 1993. Reframing policy discourse. In *The Argumentative Turn in Policy Analysis and Planning*, Eds F. Fischer and J. Forester, London, UCL Press.

Rigshospitalet. 2017. *Information and Guidance for involuntarily childless. IVF treatment.* Available at: https://www.rigshospitalet.dk/afdelinger-og-klinikker/julianemarie/fertilitetsafdelingen/undersoegelse-og-behandling/Fertilitetsbehandling/Documents/IVF%20vejledning%202017.pdf

Roberts, B. 2002. *Biographical Research*, Buckingham, Open University Press.

Rose, N. 2001. The politics of life itself, *Theory, Culture & Society*, 18(6), 1–30.

Rose, N. 2003. At regere friheden: En analyse af politisk magt i avanceret liberale demokratier. In *Perspektiv, magt og styring: Luhmann og Foucault til diskussion*, Eds C. Borch and L.L. Thorup, pp. 180–200, Copenhagen, Hans Reitzels Forlag.

Rose, N. 2007. *Politics of Life Itself: Biomedicine, Power and Subjectivity in the Twenty-First Century*, Princeton, NJ, Princeton University Press.

Rose, N., O'Malley, P. and Valverde, M. 2006. Governmentality, *Annual Review of Law and Social Science*, 2(1), 83–104.

Rose, S. 1997. *Lifelines. Life beyond the Gene*, New York, NY, Oxford University Press.

Rosenbeck, B. 1995. Pro et Contra. In *Forplantning, køn og teknologi*, Eds B. Rosenbeck and R.M. Scott, Copenhagen, Museum Tusculanums Forlag.

Roseneil, S. 2006. The ambivalences of Angel's 'arrangement': a psychosocial lens on the contemporary condition of personal life, *The Sociological Review*, 54(4), 847–869.

Rosenthal, G. 1993. Reconstruction of life stories: principles of selection in generating stories for narrative biographical interviews, *The Narrative Study of Lives*, 1(1), 59–91. [online] Available at: http://nbn-resolving.de/urn:nbn:de:0168-ssoar-59294

Rosenthal, G. 2004. Biographical research. In *Qualitative Research Practice*, Eds G. Gobo, J. Gubrium, C. Seale, and D. Silverman, London, SAGE.

Salomon, M., et al. 2015. Sociodemographic characteristics and attitudes towards motherhood among single women compared with cohabiting women treated with donor semen – a Danish multicenter study, *Acta Obstetricia et Gynecologica Scandinavica*, 94(5), 473–481.

Sauer, B. 2010. Framing and gendering. In *Politics of State Feminism: Innovation in Comparative Research*, Eds D.E. McBride and A.G. Mazur, pp. 193–216, Philadelphia, PA, Temple University Press.

Scheib, J.E., et al. 2005. Adolescents with open-identity sperm donors: reports from 12-17 year olds, *Human Reproduction*, 20(1), 239–252.

Schmidt, L. 2006. Infertility and assisted reproduction in Denmark. Epidemiology and psychosocial consequences. *Danish Medical Bulletin*, 4(53), 390–417.

Schmidt, L. 2010. Should men and women be encouraged to start childbearing at a younger age? *Expert Reviews of Obstetrics & Gynecology*, 5(2), 145–147.

Schmidt, L. and Sejrbæk, C.S. 2012. Psychosocial consequences of infertility and fertility treatment, *Ugeskrift for Læger (Danish Medical Journal)*, 174(41), 2459–2462.

Schmidt, L. and Ziebe, S. 2013. Diskussion om burgerbetaling for assisteret befrugtning. In *Danish Council of Ethics. Etik og Prioritering i sundhedsvæsnet – hvorfor er det så svært?* pp. 97–103, Copenhagen, Danish Council of Ethics.

Schön, D. and Rein, M. 1994. *Frame Reflection: Towards the Resolution of Intractable Policy Controversies*, New York, NY, Basic Books.

Schultz-Jørgensen, P. and Christensen, R.S. 2011. Den fleksible familie. In *Små og store forandringer: Danskernes værdier siden 1981*, Ed. P. Gundelach, Copenhagen, Hans Reitzels Forlag.

Scott, C.L., Wilder, S., Bennett, J. 2019. Going it alone: a multigenerational investigation of women's perceptions of single mothers by choice versus circumstance. In *Childbearing and the Changing Nature of Parenthood: The Contexts, Actors, and Experiences of Having Children (Contemporary Perspectives in Family Research*, Eds R.P. Costa and S.L. Blair, pp. 143–164, Vol. 14, Emerald Publishing Limited.

Sevón, E. 2005. Timing motherhood: experiencing and narrating the choice to become a mother, *Feminism and Psychology*, 15(4), 461–482.

Shenfield, F., de Mouzon, J., Pennings, G., Ferraretti, A.P., Andersen, A.N., de Wert, G., Goossens, V. and The ESHRE Taskforce on Cross Border Reproductive Care. 2010. Cross border reproductive care in six European countries, *Human Reproduction*, 25(6), 1361–1368.

Silva, E.B. and Smart, C. 1998. The 'new' practises and politics of family life. In *The New Family?* Eds E. Silva and C. Smart, pp. 1–13, London, Sage Publications.

Sobotka, T. 2008. Overview chapter 6: the diverse faces of the second demographic transition, *Demographic Research*, 19(8), 171–224.

Sobotka, T. and Toulemon, L. 2008. Overview chapter 4: changing family and partnership behavior: common trends and persistent diversity, *Demographic Research*, 19(6), 85–138.

Sobotka, T., Hansen, M.A., Jensen, T.K., Pedersen, A.T., Lutz, W. and Skakkebæk, N.E. 2008. The contribution of assisted reproduction to completed fertility: an analysis of Danish data, *Population and Development Review*, 34(1), 79–101.

Statistics Denmark. 2017. *Vital Statistics 2017*. [online], Copenhagen, Statistics Denmark. Available at: https://www.dst.dk/Site/Dst/Udgivelser/GetPubFile.aspx?id=22259&sid=staa

Statistics Denmark. 2019. *The Rainbow Family Has Grown*, Copenhagen, Statistics Denmark. Available at: https://www.dst.dk/da/Statistik/bagtal/2019/2019-08-14-regnbuefamilien-er-blevet-stoerre

Statistics Denmark. 2020a. *Divorces*, Copenhagen, Statistics Denmark. Available at: https://www.dst.dk/da/Statistik/emner/befolkning-og-valg/vielser-og-skilsmisser/skilsmisser

Statistics Denmark. 2020b. Marriages and divorces 2019. *Nyt fra Danmarks Statistik*, 50, 13. February. [pdf] Copenhagen: Statistics Denmark. Available at: https://www.dst.dk/Site/Dst/Udgivelser/nyt/GetPdf.aspx?cid=30085

Statistics Denmark. 2020c. *Vital Statistics 2019*, Copenhagen, Statistics Denmark. Available at: https://www.dst.dk/Site/Dst/Udgivelser/GetPubFile.aspx?id=29444 &sid=befudv2019

Statistics Denmark. 2020d. *Fertility Has Decreased to 1.7 Child Per Women*, Copenhagen, Statistics Denmark. Available at: https://www.dst.dk/Site/Dst/Udgivelser/nyt/GetPdf.aspx?cid=30330

The British Human Fertilisation & Embryology Authority (HFEA). 2020a. Fertility treatment 2018: trends and figures. Available at: https://www.hfea.gov.uk/about-us/publications/research-and-data/fertility-treatment-2018-trends-and-figures/

The British Human Fertilisation & Embryology Authority (HFEA). 2020b. Risks of fertility treatment. Available at: https://www.hfea.gov.uk/treatments/explore-all-treatments/risks-of-fertility-treatment/

The Danish Council of Ethics. 2004. *Kunstig befrugtning - etisk Set.* [pdf], Copenhagen, The Danish Council of Ethics. Available at: http://www.etiskraad.dk/~/media/Etisk-Raad/Etiske-Temaer/Assisteret-reproduktion/Publikationer/2004-01-04-kunstig-befrugtning-etisk-set.pdf

The Danish Council of Ethics. 2010. *Etiske aspekter ved nye typer af stamceller og befrugtningsteknikker*, [pdf] Copenhagen, The Danish Council of Ethics. Available at: http://www.etiskraad.dk/~/media/Etisk-Raad/Etiske-Temaer/Stamceller/Publikationer/Etiske-aspekter-ved-nye-typer-af-stamceller-og-befrugtningsteknikker.pdf

The Danish Health Data Authority. 2020. *Assisted Reproduction 2018*, Copenhagen, The Danish Health Data Authority.

Thørnhøj-Thomsen, T. 1998. *Tilblivelseshistorier: barnløshed, slægtskab og forplantningsteknologi i Danmark*, Ph. D. -række, nr. 12 1999, Kbh, Københavns Universitet Institut for Antropologi, 283 s.

Thompson, C. 2005. *Making Parents: The Ontological Choreography of Reproductive Technologies*, Cambridge, MA, The MIT Press.

Thomsen, T.L. 2005. *Immigrant Entrepreneurship as Gendered Social Positions – A Study on Motivations and Strategies in a Biographical Perspective.* PhD. AMID, Academy for Migration Studies in Denmark, Aalborg University.

Throsby, K. 2004. Normalising IVF: negotiating nature and technology. In *When IVF Fails: Feminism, Infertility, and the Negotiation of Normality*, Ed. K. Throsby, pp. 54–79, London, Palgrave Macmillan.

Tjørnhøj-Thomsen 1999. *Tilblivelseshistorier: Barnløshed, slægtskab og forplantningsteknologi i Danmark*. PhD University of Copenhage: Department of Anthropology.

Tjørnhøj-Thomsen, L. 2003. Børns sociale og kulturelle betydninger: Et barnløst perspektiv på børn, *Barn*, 1, 63–81.

Verhaak, C.M., et al. 2007. Women's emotional adjustment to IVF: a systematic review of 25 years of research, *Human Reproduction Update*, 13(1), 27–36.

Volgsten, H. and Schmidt, L. 2019. Motherhood through medically assisted reproduction - characteristics and motivations of Swedish single mothers by choice, *Human Fertility*.

Wagenaar, H. 2011. *Meaning in Action: Interpretation and Dialogue in Policy Analysis*, London, M.E. Sharpe.

Waldby, C. and Cooper, M. 2008. The biopolitics of reproduction. *Australian Feminist Studies*, 23(55), 57–73.

Wang, J. and Sauer, M.V. 2006. In vitro fertilization (IVF): a review of 3 decades of clinical innovation and technological advancement, *Therapeutics and Clinical Risk Management*, 2(4), 355–364.

Weinraub, M., Horvath, D.L. and Gringlas, M.B. 2002. Single parenthood. In *Handbook of Parenting, Vol III. Being and Becoming a Parent*, Ed. M.H. Bornstein, pp. 109–140, London, Lawrence Erlbaum Associates.

Weissenberg, R., et al. 2007. Older single mothers assisted by sperm donation and their children. *Human Reproduction*, 22(10), 2784–2791.

Wengraf, T. 2001. Qualitative research interviewing. *Biographic Narrative and Semi-Structured Methods*, London, Sage Publications.

Woollet, A. and Boyle, M. 2000. Reproduction, women's lives and subjectivities, *Feminism & Psychology*, 10(3), 307–311.

Zadeh, S., et al. 2017. Children's thoughts and feelings about their donor and security of attachment to their solo mothers in middle childhood, *Human Reproduction*, 32(4), 868–875.

Zadeh, S., et al. 2015. Absence of presence? Complexities in the donor narratives of single mothers using sperm donation, *Human Reproduction*, 31(1), 1–8.

Zadeh, S., Freeman, T., and Golombok, S. 2013. Ambivalent identities of single women using sperm donation. *Revue internationale de Psychologie Sociale-International Review of Social Psychology*, 26(3), 97–123.

Zegers-Hochschild, F., et al. 2009. The international committee for monitoring assisted reproductive technology (ICMART) and the World Health Organization (WHO) revised glossary on ART terminology, *Human Reproduction*, 24(11), 2683–2687.

Zegers-Hochschild, F., et al. 2017. The international glossary on infertility and fertility care, *Human Reproduction*, 32(9), 1786–1801.

Index